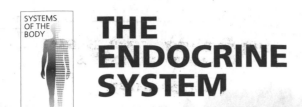

SYSTEMS
OF THE
BODY

THE
ENDOCRINE
SYSTEM

This book is dedicated to the memory of
Dr Saad Al-Damluji, endocrinologist
and teacher.

SYSTEMS
OF THE
BODY

Commissioning Editor: Michael Parkinson
Development Editor: Lulu Stader
Project Manager: Emma Riley
Designer: Erik Bigland
Illustraton Buyer: Gillian Richards
Illustrator: Robert Britton

THE ENDOCRINE SYSTEM

Joy Hinson BSc PhD DSc

Reader in Molecular and Cellular Endocrinology, Dean for Postgraduate Studies, Barts and The London, Queen Mary's School of Medicine and Dentistry, London, UK

Peter Raven BSc PhD MBBS MRCP MRCPsych FHEA

Faculty Tutor (Biomedical Sciences), UCL, Director, Metabolic and Clinical Trials Unit, Royal Free and University College Medical School, UCL & Honorary Consultant Psychiatrist, Camden and Islington Mental Health Trust, London, UK

Shern Chew BSc MD FRCP

Professor of Endocrine Medicine/Consultant Physician, Barts and the London, Queen Mary's School of Medicine and Dentistry, London, UK

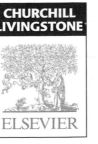

CHURCHILL LIVINGSTONE

ELSEVIER

EDINBURGH LONDON NEW YORK OXFORD PHILADELPHIA ST LOUIS SYDNEY TORONTO 2007

CHURCHILL
LIVINGSTONE
ELSEVIER

First published 2007

ISBN: 978-0-443-06237-7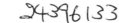

British Library Cataloguing in Publication Data
A catalogue record for this book is available from the British Library

Library of Congress Cataloging in Publication Data
A catalog record for this book is available from the Library of Congress

Notice
Knowledge and best practice in this field are constantly changing. As new research and experience broaden our knowledge, changes in practice, treatment and drug therapy may become necessary or appropriate. Readers are advised to check the most current information provided (i) on procedures featured or (ii) by the manufacturer of each product to be administered, to verify the recommended dose or formula, the method and duration of administration, and contraindications. It is the responsibility of the practitioner, relying on their own experience and knowledge of the patient, to make diagnoses, to determine dosages and the best treatment for each individual patient, and to take all appropriate safety precautions. To the fullest extent of the law, neither the Publisher nor the Authors assume any liability for any injury and/ or damage to persons or property arising out or related to any use of the material contained in this book.

The Publisher

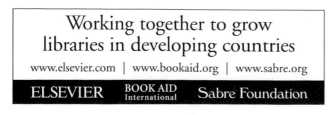
Printed in Europe

'Endocrinology is really very simple. You can either have too much of a hormone … or too little.'
(Professor John Landon's traditional and reassuring introduction to his endocrinology teaching.)

This book is aimed at medical students, particularly those taking a modern integrated course. By structuring each chapter around a clinical case, our intention is to allow medical students early in their studies to understand the clinical relevance of the basic science. But we also hope that the book will act as an explanation of the basic science underlying endocrine disease for students during their clinical studies.

The book is intended as an introduction to the Endocrine System, although we hope that you will be sufficiently enthused after reading it to wish to take your studies further in this exciting area.

In the clinical cases featured in this book we have tried to show common presentations of the different disorders, but endocrine problems present in such a wide variety of ways that students should not be misled into thinking that these are the only presentations! Throughout the book we have included *Interesting Facts*: these are snippets of information that particularly interested us and that we wanted to share with you. We hope that you find them interesting too.

Chapters 1 and 11 are not case-based. Chapter 1 contains the basic concepts needed to understand the endocrine system, and Chapter 11 contains a mixture of hormones and signalling molecules with varying degrees of clinical importance. This last chapter illustrates perfectly the idea that endocrinology is rather more than a stand-alone speciality and impinges on the cardiovascular system, the immune system and all other systems of the body.

We do hope that we have managed to convey to you our enthusiasm for this most fascinating subject.

Joy Hinson, Peter Raven, Shern Chew
London 2006

ACKNOWLEDGEMENTS

We are most grateful to all our colleagues for their help and advice in the preparation of this book. In particular we would like to thank: Dr Dan Berney for providing the histology, Dr Norbert Avril for the whole-body glucose image and Dr Alistair Chesser for the EPO case. Thanks also to Dr Antonia Brooke, Derek and Niloufar (you know why), Dr John Patterson and Mrs Jacqualyn Conner. Although many colleagues have helped and advised us, all errors remain our own.

Thanks are due also to the team at Elsevier led by Mike Parkinson, and especially to our editor, Lulu Stader. Without Lulu's encouragement we would never have got this far. We'll miss the daily e-mails, hourly phone calls and the pictures of your garden.

CONTENTS

INTRODUCTION

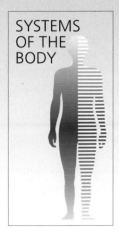

SYSTEMS OF THE BODY

Chapter objectives

After reading this chapter you should be able to:

① Understand that hormones exert their effects by binding to specific receptors in target tissues.

② Categorize common hormones by their basic chemical structures and the types of receptor they bind to.

③ Understand the role of plasma binding proteins for some hormones.

④ Understand the different forms of endocrine regulation, including set point, diurnal variation, endocrine axis and negative feedback.

⑤ Understand the basis of endocrine disease.

⑥ Appreciate the purpose and types of endocrine testing.

What is endocrinology?

Endocrinology is the study of hormones and their actions. Hormones are chemical messengers, released into the blood, that act through receptors to cause a change in the target cell. The glands that release hormones are ductless, giving the term 'endocrine' from the Greek for 'internal secretion'. The thyroid gland is an example of a classical endocrine gland. Its only function is to synthesize and release hormones into the bloodstream. Some organs, such as the pancreas, have endocrine as well as other functions. So the hormones released by the pancreas are released directly into the blood, whereas the other (exocrine) secretions of the pancreas are released into a duct.

The major, or 'classical', endocrine glands are shown in Figure 1.1. It has been suggested that the vascular epithelium, the whole gastrointestinal tract, and even the skin, should also be considered to be endocrine organs as they all release hormones or their precursors into the blood. Such tissues form the extensive 'diffuse endocrine system' which is located throughout the body. This system consists of scattered endocrine cells, located in various different tissues, that secrete hormones but do not form a discrete endocrine gland.

Endocrinology is a relatively young branch of medical science and is, by definition, exciting. The term 'hormone' was coined by Starling in the early 1900s. It derives from the Greek 'hormon', meaning 'exciting' or 'setting in motion'. Ernest Starling (1866–1927) is perhaps best known for his eponymous law of the cardiovascular system, but is also regarded as the founder of endocrinology. Working at University College, London, with Sir William Bayliss, he isolated and described the actions of secretin, the first known hormone. Starling built on the theoretical work of Edward Schafer and developed the concept of 'an endocrine system' in 1905, in a series of lectures called 'On the chemical correlations of the functions of the body'.

Interesting fact

2005 saw the centenary of Endocrinology as a recognized science and branch of medicine. Learned societies, such as the Society for Endocrinology, have celebrated this with a series of special published articles, lectures, events and poster campaigns (Fig. 1.2). To put this into perspective, surgery and pharmacology have been around for thousands of years.

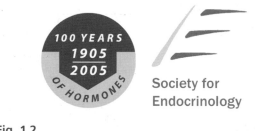

Fig. 1.2
In 2005 the Society for Endocrinology celebrated the centenary of Endocrinology as a recognized science.

Endocrine regulation

Hormones usually control regulatory systems in the body, including homeostasis, metabolism and reproduction. Neural regulation is very rapid, but endocrine control is generally slower and acts over a longer period of time. The boundaries between the endocrine system and the neural system are quite fuzzy (Fig. 1.3), because some hormones are released from nerve endings, 'neurohormones', while other hormones, such as adrenaline, are perhaps better known as neurotransmitters.

Types of hormone: their synthesis and secretion

In terms of their chemical structure, hormones are a varied group of substances. There are, however, three basic types. The first and most numerous are the

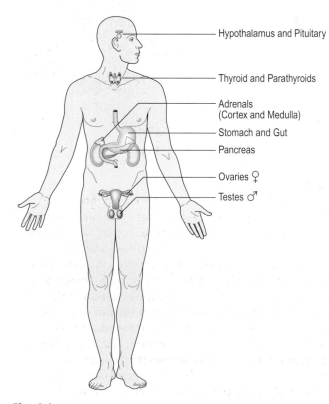

- Hypothalamus and Pituitary
- Thyroid and Parathyroids
- Adrenals (Cortex and Medulla)
- Stomach and Gut
- Pancreas
- Ovaries ♀
- Testes ♂

Fig. 1.1
Major endocrine glands of the body. In addition, the gut, heart and skin have all been shown to produce hormones.

peptide hormones, made of chains of amino acids. Some of these are very small indeed: the hypothalamic hormone thyrotropin releasing hormone (TRH) is only three amino acids long, whereas the pituitary hormone whose release it stimulates (thyroid stimulating hormone, TSH) is a large glycoprotein with a molecular weight of around 30 000 daltons. Usually, peptide hormones are pre-formed and stored in granules within the endocrine cell, ready for release in response to the appropriate signal. The synthesis and secretion of peptide hormones is shown in Figure 1.4A.

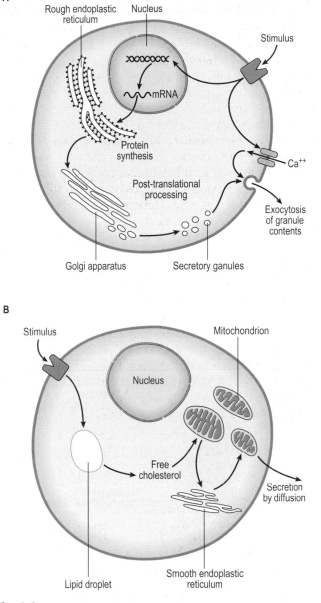

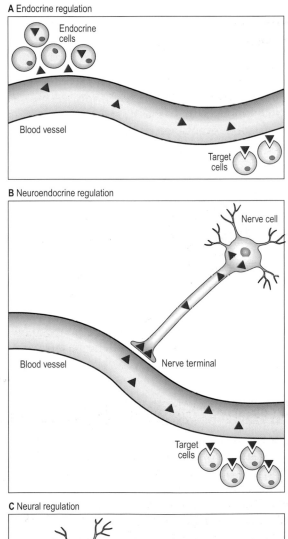

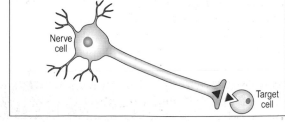

Fig. 1.3
Comparison of (A) endocrine, (B) neuroendocrine and (C) neural regulation.

Fig. 1.4
Synthesis and secretion of (A) peptide hormones and (B) steroid hormones. The cells that synthesize peptide hormones have abundant rough endoplasmic reticulum and Golgi apparatus. Secretory granules are often visible. Peptides require a specific secretory mechanism, exocytosis, which is usually triggered by an increase in intracellular calcium levels, or depolarization of the cell. The entire contents of the secretory granule are released. Steroid-secreting cells, on the other hand, have lipid droplets visible in the cytoplasm. They have abundant mitochondria and smooth endoplasmic reticulum. The steroid hormones, once made, simply diffuse out of the cell and do not require a specific secretory mechanism.

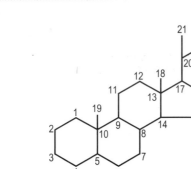

Fig. 1.5

Structure of cholesterol, the parent compound for all steroid hormones and vitamin D. The classical steroid system for numbering carbon atoms is shown.

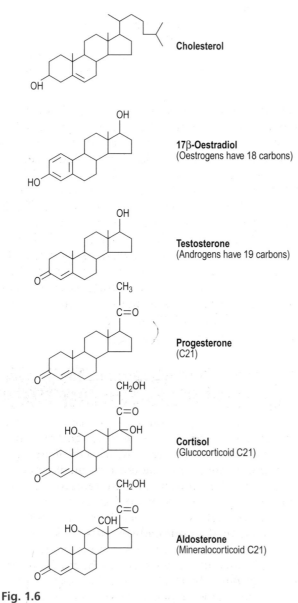

Cholesterol

17β-Oestradiol
(Oestrogens have 18 carbons)

Testosterone
(Androgens have 19 carbons)

Progesterone
(C21)

Cortisol
(Glucocorticoid C21)

Aldosterone
(Mineralocorticoid C21)

Fig. 1.6

The major families of steroid hormones.

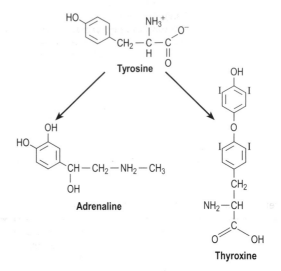

Tyrosine

Adrenaline

Thyroxine

Fig. 1.7

Metabolism of the amino acid tyrosine produces both thyroid hormones (thyroxine) and catecholamines (adrenaline).

The second major group of hormones consists of the steroids. These are all made from cholesterol (Fig. 1.4B) and have a common core structure (Fig. 1.5). Quite small chemical changes to this core structure cause significant differences in their biological effects (Fig. 1.6). The pathways of steroid hormone biosynthesis are shown in the adrenal chapter and the chapters on reproduction.

The third group of hormones are those derived from amino acids. For example, tyrosine residues can be iodinated to give thyroid hormones, or hydroxylated as the first step on the biosynthetic pathway of the catecholamines: dopamine, adrenaline and noradrenaline (Fig. 1.7). A detailed account of the synthesis of thyroid hormones in given in Chapter 5.

The differences in chemical structure of hormones have implications for the way in which these hormones are made, their mechanism of action and, of course, their route of administration (Table 1.1). For example, steroid hormones and thyroid hormones are orally active, whereas most peptide hormones (such as insulin) must be injected, to avoid being inactivated by digestive enzymes, if they are used therapeutically. Most endocrine cells have stores of hormone that can be released as soon as they are needed. While peptide hormones are synthesized then stored in granules in the cells (see Fig. 1.4A), steroid-secreting cells keep a store of cholesterol, the substrate for steroid biosynthesis, rather than the final steroid product (see Fig. 1.4B). This is largely a matter of practicality as the steroid hormones, being lipid soluble, are difficult to store, whereas cholesterol can be esterified and stored easily. Similarly, in the thyroid gland, a store of precursor

Table 1.1
Comparison of steroids, peptides, thyroid hormones and catecholamines

	Location of receptors	Carrier protein	Active if administered orally?	Synthesis
Peptides	Cell membrane	No	Not usually	Hormone stored
Steroids	Cytoplasm/nucleus	Yes	Yes, mostly	Precursor stored
Thyroid hormones	Cytoplasm/nucleus	Yes	Yes	Precursor stored
Catecholamines	Cell membrane	No	No	Hormone stored

Table 1.2
Concentrations of various substances in blood

Substance	Concentration in SI units (using conventional abbreviations)	Log mol/L and equivalent SI unit (per litre) in full	
Sodium	140 mmol/L	10^{-1}	100 millimoles
Bicarbonate	21–26 mmol/L	10^{-2}	10 millimoles
Glucose	3–5 mmol/L	10^{-3}	1 millimole
Uric acid	150–500 µmol/L	10^{-4}	100 micromoles
Iron	10–30 µmol/L	10^{-5}	10 micromoles
Vitamin A	0.5–2 µmol/L	10^{-6}	1 micromole
Cortisol (9 am)	200–650 nmol/L	10^{-7}	100 nanomoles
Testosterone (men)	10–35 nmol/L	10^{-8}	10 nanomoles
Tri-iodothyronine	1–3.5 nmol/L	10^{-9}	1 nanomole
Adrenaline (resting)	170–500 pmol/L	10^{-10}	100 picomoles
Free thyroxine	10–30 pmol/L	10^{-11}	10 picomoles
Oxytocin (basal)	1–4 pmol/L	10^{-12}	1 picomole

Table 1.3
Hormones and their binding proteins

Hormone	Binding protein
Thyroid hormone	Thyroid hormone binding globulin (THBG)
Testosterone/oestradiol	Sex hormone binding globulin (SHBG)
Cortisol	Cortisol binding globulin (CBG, also called transcortin)
Vitamin D	Vitamin D binding protein (DBP)

is maintained, from which thyroid hormones may be readily released.

As a consequence of their small and lipophilic nature, steroid hormones do not require a specific secretory mechanism: they simply diffuse across the plasma membrane and out of the cell down a concentration gradient. Peptide hormones, on the other hand, need a specific secretory mechanism (see Fig. 1.4).

Hormones in blood

Hormones circulate in blood in very low concentrations indeed, and for this reason they are measured in units that are unfamiliar to many people (Table 1.2). Although some hormones, mostly the peptide hormones, are freely water-soluble, the steroid and thyroid hormones are not so soluble, and need to be transported in blood bound to a carrier or binding protein (Table 1.3). Not all steroids have a specific binding protein: aldosterone, for example, does not have a specific carrier protein, and circulates in blood bound mostly to albumin. The binding proteins have three

main functions. First, they increase the solubility of the hormone in blood. Second, they increase the biological half-life of the hormone by protecting it from metabolism and excretion, so that aldosterone, which does not have a carrier protein, has a half-life of around 15 minutes, whereas cortisol, which is bound to cortisol binding globulin (CBG), has a half-life of 90 minutes. Third, the binding proteins create a readily accessible reserve of the hormone in blood. Only the fraction of hormone that is not bound to the carrier protein is considered to be biologically active. This is one factor that must be considered when measuring circulating concentrations of hormones. It is particularly important because levels of binding proteins can be altered in some clinical conditions and by some drugs.

Different mechanisms of action of hormones

All hormones act by binding to receptors in their target cells and so initiating an intracellular response. It is the presence of receptors, which are highly specific binding proteins, that determines the target cells for a hormone. The location of these receptors in each cell depends to some extent on the chemical nature of the hormone (Table 1.4). Steroids and thyroid hormones, being small and lipophilic, pass readily across the cell membrane and classically bind to intracellular receptors, located in the nucleus. The hormone-receptor complex binds to DNA, to specific response elements in the promoter region of specific genes, and stimulates gene transcription. In this way, steroid and

Table 1.4
Classification of hormone receptors

Structure	Agonist/ ligand	Signalling mechanism
Plasma membrane: seven-transmembrane domain	Multiple types of ligand: peptides, catecholamines	G-protein/second messenger activating kinase
Plasma membrane: single-transmembrane domain	Large peptides: growth factors, cytokines	Kinase cascade
Nuclear	Lipophilic hormones: steroids, thyroid hormone, calcitriol (vitamin D3)	Binds to DNA and activates/ suppresses gene transcription

thyroid hormones increase the production of certain proteins and thereby alter cellular function (Fig. 1.9).

Peptides, glycoproteins and catecholamines, on the other hand, are either too large or too hydrophilic to enter the cell and so these hormones bind to receptors located in the plasma membrane, with their ligand binding domain on the extracellular surface. There are four broad classes of cell surface receptor. The first group is the seven-transmembrane domain receptors, which are linked to G-protein activation and to second messenger production or ion channel opening (Fig. 1.10). The major second messenger systems and' the kinases they activate are shown in Figure 1.11.

All of the other groups are single-transmembrane domain receptors, which may be found as either single units or homodimers. The second group comprises the family of single-transmembrane domain receptors that function as dimers. These receptors possess inherent tyrosine kinase activity and activate a kinase cascade (Fig. 1.12A). The third group, which have only recently been characterized, are single-transmembrane domain receptors that do not have inherent kinase activity, but that dimerize after binding and thus activate the Janus-associated kinase–signal transducer and activator of transcription (JAK–STAT) pathway (Fig. 1.12B). The fourth group consists of a single transmembrane receptor possessing guanylate cyclase activity and acting through cyclic guanosine monophosphate (cGMP) generation (Fig. 1.12C).

In each case there is ultimately phosphorylation of proteins, which are usually enzymes; this either activates or inactivates the enzyme, thus bringing about a change in cellular function. Examples of hormones acting through these different types of receptor are given in Table 1.5. The phosphorylated proteins often

Interesting fact

Classically, hormones travel from the cells where they are made, in the bloodstream, to reach the cells where they act. But some hormones also act locally, on different cell types in the tissue where they are produced. This is termed a 'paracrine' effect. Other hormones act directly on the same type of cell that secretes them. This is termed an 'autocrine' action (Fig. 1.8). Hormones may have a mixture of different types of action. An example of this is testosterone, which exerts a paracrine effect on spermatogenesis in the testis, but an endocrine effect on other tissues.

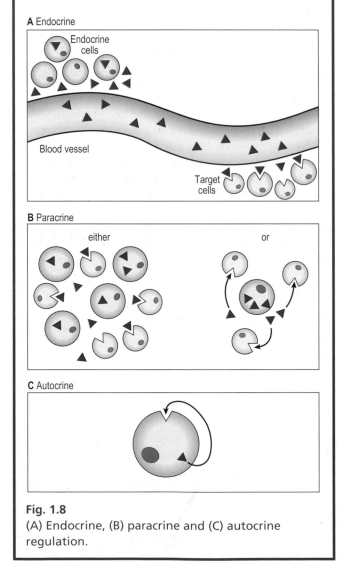

Fig. 1.8
(A) Endocrine, (B) paracrine and (C) autocrine regulation.

form 'kinase cascades'. There are several examples of these, for example the family of mitogen-activated protein kinase (MAPK) cascade involved in cell division (Fig. 1.13).

INTRODUCTION

1

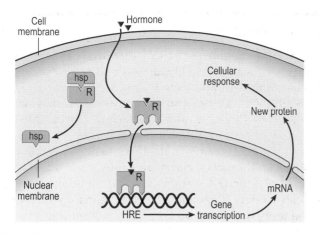

Fig. 1.9

Mechanism of steroid hormone action. Receptors for steroid hormones are found inside the cell, in either the cytoplasm or the nucleus. In the resting state, these receptors are associated with proteins called heat shock proteins (hsp). The steroid crosses the cell membrane and binds to the receptor, displacing the hsp. The hormone–receptor complex is then able to pass into the nucleus and bind to hormone response elements (HREs) in the promoter region of certain genes. This can activate or repress transcription of that gene, causing changes in mRNA and therefore new protein formation in the cell.

Endocrine regulation

The endocrine system is involved in a variety of homeostatic mechanisms in the body. In many cases regulation involves maintenance of a 'set point' and correction of any deviation from this point. One example is the regulation of plasma calcium concentration, which is tightly controlled within close set limits. In this case, any deviation from the set point triggers a hormonal response which acts to correct the calcium level (see Chapter 10).

The concentrations of some hormones are also maintained at a set point, for example thyroxine, whereas others vary more widely, for example growth hormone. This wide variation may be due to both diurnal variation or in response to physiological demand. Such hormones are said to be secreted 'episodically' (Fig. 1.14).

Diurnal variation

The secretion of many hormones has a predictable daily pattern (see Fig. 1.14). Growth hormone concentrations, for example, are usually so low that they are undetectable during the day, but increase during the early part of sleep. In contrast, corticotropin concentrations are at their lowest at midnight and reach a peak at around 8 am each day. It is clearly important to be aware of diurnal variation when circulating hormone levels are being measured.

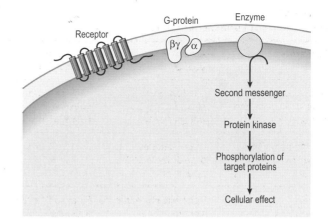

Fig. 1.10

Peptide hormone action 1: hormone action through a G-protein-coupled receptor. The receptors are a family of similar proteins located in the plasma membrane of the target cell. They are all folded to give a similar conformation, with seven regions that span the membrane, and so are sometime called 'seven-transmembrane domain receptors'. The receptors are linked to membrane proteins called G-proteins, which carry the signal from the receptor to an enzyme that makes second messengers. There are several 'families' of G-proteins involved in signal transduction. The proteins have three subunits, termed α, β and γ. In each case it is the α subunit that differs and makes the G-protein specific for an enzyme. G-protein activation of an enzyme or ion channel causes an increase in intracellular content of a 'second messenger' chemical, which binds to a specific protein kinase, activating it and causing phosphorylation of certain proteins, and leading to a change in cellular activity.

> **Interesting fact**
>
> Although the major 'classical' actions of steroids are mediated by nuclear receptors, it is increasingly recognized that steroids can also act through plasma membrane receptors. It is activation of these receptors that accounts for the rapid actions of some steroids, first postulated by Hans Selye in the 1940s, when it was shown that certain steroids can act as anaesthetics.

Endocrine axis

Many hormones function as part of a cascade, so that the target tissue of one hormone is another endocrine gland. For example, thyrotropin releasing hormone (TRH) from the hypothalamus stimulates the release of pituitary TSH, which in turn stimulates release of T4 from the thyroid. The cascade allows amplifications

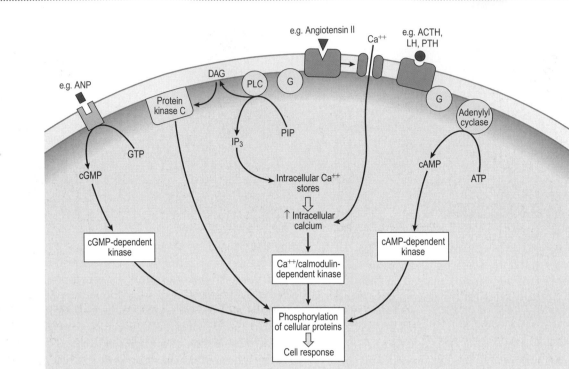

Fig. 1.11
Second messenger systems involved in endocrine signalling. Hormones acting through a receptor linked to adenylyl cyclase exert their effect through an increase in intracellular cyclic adenosine monophosphate (cAMP) levels. There are many examples of hormones that act through cAMP generation. A less common mechanism of action is through a receptor linked to phospholipase C (PLC). Activation of this enzyme causes cleavage of the membrane phospholipids, phosphatidylinositolbisphosphate (PIP$_2$), to release inositol trisphosphate (IP$_3$) and diacylglycerol (DAG). The DAG activates protein kinase C. The IP$_3$ acts on intracellular organelles such as the endoplasmic reticulum, to release intracellular stores of calcium. The increase in intracellular calcium concentration activates calcium/calmodulin-dependent kinase. Finally, hormones acting through a receptor with intrinsic guanylyl cyclase activity, such as the atrial natriuretic peptide (ANP) receptor, cause intracellular levels of cGMP to increase, activating the cGMP-dependent kinase. It can be seen that activation of each second messenger pathway results in the activation of a kinase, allowing phosphorylation of cellular proteins and so bringing about the cellular response. ACTH, adrenocorticotropic hormone; G, G-protein; LH, luteinizing hormone; PTH, parathyroid hormone.

of signal, flexibility of response to a variety of physiological stimuli and fine regulation of levels of the end hormonal product. This functional grouping is called an endocrine axis (Fig. 1.15) and in the example we have used is called the hypothalamo–pituitary–thyroid axis.

Negative feedback
One of the most important principles of endocrine regulation is the concept of negative feedback. This form of regulation is where the final product of an endocrine cascade acts to inhibit release of hormones higher up the cascade (see Fig. 1.15). The hormones that exert this form of negative feedback effect are usually small molecules that can cross the blood–brain barrier, as the hypothalamus is an important site of negative feedback in many hormone systems.

The principle of negative feedback is the basis of several dynamic tests of endocrine function. This form of regulation is covered in more detail in Chapter 3.

Endocrine disorders and investigations of endocrine function

As a general rule, endocrine disorders are the result of either excessive secretion of a hormone or of insufficient secretion. The effects of either hormone excess or relative absence of hormone are exaggerations of the normal physiological effects of the hormone and serve as a very useful illustration of endocrine physiology. Historically endocrine disease states were used to gain an understanding of the actions of different hormones. The cases used in this book have been

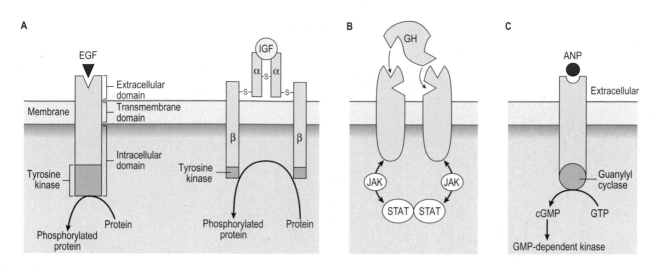

Fig. 1.12

Peptide hormone action 2. (A) Hormone action through a growth factor receptor, with intrinsic tyrosine kinase activity. The receptor is either a single transmembrane unit such as the epidermal growth factor (EGF) receptor, or a homodimer such as the insulin or insulin-like growth factor (IGF) receptor. The insulin receptor consists of a dimer with each part having an α and β subunit. The whole receptor is held together by disulphide bridges, indicated as –s– in the diagram. When the hormone binds to the receptor it causes a conformational change within the receptor which activates the protein tyrosine kinase, resulting in the direct phosphorylation of intracellular proteins. (B) Hormone action through a cytokine receptor (or growth hormone [GH] receptor). Binding of the hormone to the first receptor causes a conformational change which allows the receptor to dimerize and the hormone to bind to the second receptor subunit; in this case the conformational change in the receptor causes the Janus-associated kinase (JAK) to migrate to the receptor, become activated and phosphorylate signal transducer and activator of transcription (STAT) proteins. (C) Receptor with intrinsic guanylyl cyclase activity. Formation of cGMP leads to activation of kinase pathways and protein phosphorylation. ANP, atrial natriuretic peptide. In all cases activation of a kinase pathway leads to phosphorylation of cellular proteins. These phosphorylated proteins are usually enzymes that are activated as a result of the phosphorylation. In this way the cellular function is altered.

Table 1.5
Cell membrane receptors

Receptor type	Signalling system	Hormones acting through this type of receptor
G-protein-coupled receptor (seven-transmembrane domain receptor)	Second messengers: cAMP	ACTH, glucagon, parathyroid hormone, TSH, etc
	Inositol trisphosphate/diacylglycerol/ calcium	Angiotensin II, oxytocin, gonadotropin releasing hormone
Single-transmembrane domain receptors		
Growth factor receptor	Receptor has inbuilt tyrosine kinase activity	Insulin, insulin-like growth factor (IGF)
Cytokine receptor	Receptor interacts with kinases such as JAK–STAT	Growth hormone, prolactin, erythropoietin
Guanylyl cyclase receptors	Receptor has inbuilt guanylyl cyclase activity; acts through generation of cGMP	ANP: atrial natriuretic peptide

chosen to illustrate important points about either the biochemistry of hormone synthesis or the physiology of endocrine regulation.

The endocrine axes described above mean that a deficiency in the final hormone of the cascade may be due to a defect at one of several points in the axis. Looking at the example of an endocrine axis shown in Figure 1.15, a defect in the thyroid gland itself would result in primary thyroid failure, a problem with pituitary secretion of TSH would be called secondary thyroid failure,

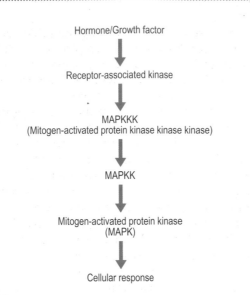

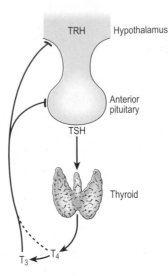

Fig. 1.13

An example of a kinase cascade: mitogen-activated protein kinase (MAPK). Each of the kinases in this cascade refers to a family of proteins, which is associated with different aspects of cellular function. For example, the MAPK family includes the kinase P38 which has a role in apoptosis, and ERK1 and ERK2 which have roles in cell growth.

Fig. 1.15

An endocrine axis and negative feedback. The axis shown is the hypothalamo–pituitary–thyroid axis. Thyrotropin releasing hormone (TRH), from the hypothalamus, stimulates the release of thyroid stimulating hormone (TSH) from the anterior pituitary. The TSH stimulates the thyroid gland to release T4 and T3, which exert a negative feedback inhibitory effect on the hypothalamus and pituitary glands.

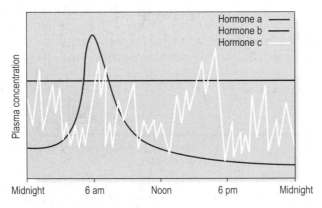

Fig. 1.14

Diurnal variation and episodic secretion. Some hormones, such as hormone a, have a pronounced diurnal variation in their secretion. An example of such a hormone would be cortisol. Other hormones such as hormone b, which could be thyroxine, show very little diurnal variation. Hormone c shows episodic secretion; this pattern is common to many different hormones. It means that taking a single-point blood measurement of the hormone is of little value in diagnosing endocrine disorder because there is so much variation during the day.

and a deficiency of TRH from the hypothalamus would be called tertiary thyroid failure.

The investigation of endocrine disorders usually starts with a simple single-point measurement of plasma hormone concentrations. In some cases this measurement may be sufficient to determine whether there is a disorder, but when the hormone under investigation is secreted episodically (such as growth hormone or cortisol) a single-point measurement is often of very limited value. In this case a *dynamic test* of the endocrine system is used. The principle of dynamic testing is really quite simple: when an excess of hormone is suspected the aim of the dynamic test is to suppress hormone levels. If, on the other hand, insufficient secretion is suspected then the aim of the test is to stimulate secretion. As far as possible the tests aim to check the whole system.

Endocrine investigations: general principles

There are two general reasons for performing endocrine investigations (Box 1.1). The first is to confirm a diagnosis and the second is to monitor the progress of a disease. There are a large number of possible tests aimed at confirming a diagnosis, and so a degree of selection and judgement has to be introduced. The selection of tests to perform must be guided by the clinical situation, and here the clinician may use two types of approach. One approach is to make a clinical diagnosis based on pattern recognition. For example, a classical combination of symptoms in endocrine disease is weight loss despite a good appetite (seen in thyrotoxicosis), which will lead an experienced clinician into testing the thyroid gland. A second approach is to use the basic principles of physiology and anatomy in guiding diagnostic testing. This is needed if the clinical pattern is unclear or a surprising result is found. For example, a patient may be found to have atrial fibrillation (an irregular heart rhythm) when undergoing a routine examination before an operation. As high thyroid hormone levels stimulate the heart, and in particular the atrial chambers, this should lead to thyroid function testing, even in the absence of other classical symptoms.

The most commonly used tests in endocrinology measure hormones and minerals in blood samples (Box 1.2). The levels of most hormones vary through the day and the normal ranges are very dependent on the time a sample is taken; thus, normal ranges are usually based on samples taken at 0900 hours and in

---

Box 1.1

Endocrine tests

- Tests may be for purposes of diagnosis or monitoring.

- Diagnostic tests may be selected after clinical pattern recognition or by understanding basic principles of physiology and anatomy.

- Blood tests may be basal or dynamic.

- Basal tests are usually at 0900 hours in a fasted state.

- In dynamic testing: select a stimulation test if a hormone level is suspected of being too low, but a suppression test if the level is suspected of being too high.

Box 1.2

Measurement of hormones

As hormones circulate in such small concentrations, measuring hormone levels in blood presents a particular challenge. Original assay methods used the biological response to a hormone to estimate the amount present and were termed 'bioassays'. An example is the early pregnancy test which relied on the observation that human chorionic gonadotropin (hCG), the level of which is raised in early pregnancy, causes the female *Xenopus* toad to ovulate. These assays had the advantage that they measured only biologically active hormone. However, they had several disadvantages: they were often relatively insensitive and they usually used animals or animal tissues. This not only raised ethical issues, but also made the assays inherently unreliable because of the variability of the response. Modern methods of hormone assay usually use a competitive binding assay, such as a radioimmunoassay, which is very sensitive (Fig. 1.16). These have been developed to a level of sophistication that makes them simple to perform, rapid and very reliable. It is now possible to purchase kits that measure all the known hormones at the concentrations found in human plasma.

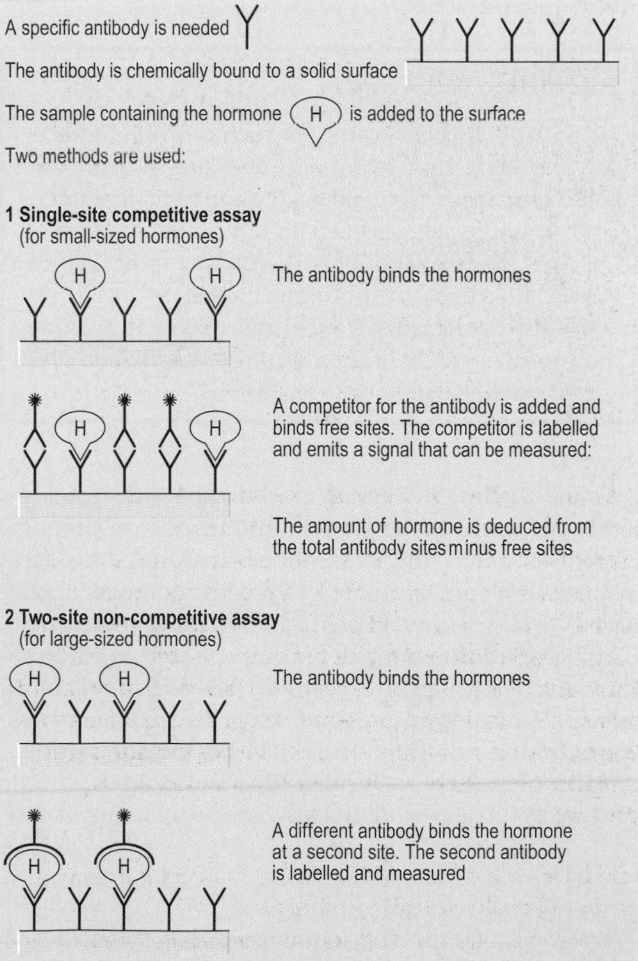

A specific antibody is needed

The antibody is chemically bound to a solid surface

The sample containing the hormone (H) is added to the surface

Two methods are used:

1 Single-site competitive assay
(for small-sized hormones)

The antibody binds the hormones

A competitor for the antibody is added and binds free sites. The competitor is labelled and emits a signal that can be measured:

The amount of hormone is deduced from the total antibody sites minus free sites

2 Two-site non-competitive assay
(for large-sized hormones)

The antibody binds the hormones

A different antibody binds the hormone at a second site. The second antibody is labelled and measured

Fig. 1.16
Measurement of hormones in blood by immunoassay.

a fasted state. It is vital to the correct interpretation of a blood test result that the time of the sample is recorded. These samples are also known as basal samples as they represent the base, or unstimulated, state. Samples are also tested at specific times after stimulation or suppression and these are called dynamic tests. An example is the stimulation of the steroid hormone cortisol from the adrenal gland 30 and 60 minutes after an injection of synthetic adrenocorticotropin.

The maximum information is obtained when a hormone and its regulator are measured together. For example, if T4 and TSH are measured together then it is immediately clear whether the disease process is in the thyroid or the pituitary.

Biological samples

All blood, urine and biopsy samples need to be collected in the correct tubes. Some hormones have a very short life and a falsely low value may occur if the procedure is not done properly. For example, adrenocorticotropin has a half-life in the blood of about 10 minutes, so the blood must be taken in a chilled syringe and bottle, and then the plasma has to be separated immediately from blood by centrifugation.

Interesting fact

Endocrine disorders can have such profound effects on the body that many disorders are 'foot of the bed' diagnoses. You will read about the characteristic changes of acromegaly, Cushing's syndrome, Graves' disease and hypothyroidism later. All of these disorders of hormone secretion result in changes to the appearance that makes it possible to recognize them from a distance. Keep your eyes open on the bus!

Urine testing is very important in endocrinology. A simple stick can be dipped into urine and chemical pads will detect the presence of glucose (suggesting diabetes), blood, protein, white cells, ketones, acidity and even hormones (e.g. hCG, indicating pregnancy). This yields a tremendous amount of clinical information and a dip-stick test should be performed in all new patients. Hormones and minerals are usually best measured in accurately timed 24-hour urine samples. All urine produced over this time is placed in a bottle and the total excretion of a hormone can be measured.

Table 1.6
Imaging and endocrine glands

Gland	Imaging modality
Pituitary and hypothalamus	Magnetic resonance imaging (MRI)
Adrenal	CT initially
Pancreas	CT initially
Thyroid	Ultrasonography
Testes	Ultrasonography
Ovaries	Ultrasonography (transvaginal)

Imaging

Radiological imaging is vital to the assessment of endocrine glands. The type of test selected depends on the gland (Table 1.6). For example, the pituitary is surrounded by a bony cup and is not well seen by radiography. The best image is obtained with magnetic resonance imaging.

Ectopic hormone secretion

It is not only the well defined endocrine tissues that can secrete hormones. All cells retain the genetic capacity for hormone secretion and it is increasingly recognized that malignant cells may express the genes encoding hormonally active peptides. As the usual mechanism for hormone processing is not usually present in these malignancies, the peptide secreted may be a fragment or a precursor of the normal mature hormone. The inappropriate secretion of hormones by tissues that do not usually produce that hormone is called 'ectopic' hormone secretion. Often ectopic hormone secretion is seen as a feature of endocrine tumours; for example, pancreatic islet cell carcinomas have occasionally been found to secrete adrenocorticotropic hormone (ACTH), which usually comes from the pituitary gland. Non-endocrine tissues may also secrete hormones; for example, inappropriate ACTH secretion is a recognized feature of some small cell carcinomas of the lung.

The most common example of ectopic hormone secretion is a peptide hormone called parathyroid hormone-related peptide (PTHrp) which is secreted by around 10% of malignant tumours and causes hypercalcaemia, termed 'hypercalcaemia of malignancy'.

Ectopic hormone secretion is diagnosed through a combined approach of imaging, together with arteriovenous sampling to measure a hormone concentration gradient across a tissue and so establish the source of the hormone.

Extended matching questions

A   Aldosterone
B   Atrial natriuretic peptide
C   Cholesterol
D   Cortisol
E   Growth hormone
F   Insulin
G   Norepinephrine (noradrenaline)
H   Prolactin
I   Testosterone
J   Thyroxine (thyroid hormone)
K   TSH (thyroid stimulating hormone)
L   Tyrosine

For each of the hormones described below, choose the name from the list above that best matches the description:

① This modified amino acid is an example of a catecholamine.

② This peptide hormone has a characteristic diurnal pattern of secretion, with undetectable levels during the day and a major secretory period during early sleep.

③ This steroid hormone is unusual in that it does not have a specific carrier protein.

④ This hormone's receptor uses cGMP as the second messenger.

⑤ This hormone is not a steroid but acts on intracellular receptors.

⑥ This hormone's receptor has a tyrosine kinase domain.

Answers see page 150

THE HYPOTHALAMUS AND PITUITARY PART I: THE HYPOTHALAMUS AND POSTERIOR PITUITARY

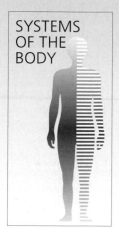

SYSTEMS OF THE BODY

Chapter objectives

After reading this chapter you should be able to:

① Describe the locations of the hypothalamus and pituitary and explain how they are connected, both anatomically and physiologically.

② Describe the hormones secreted from the posterior pituitary and outline their actions.

③ Describe how these hormones are synthesized and secreted.

④ Explain what is meant by the term 'neuroendocrine reflex'.

⑤ Describe the clinical effects of under-production of arginine vasopressin.

⑥ Explain the science underlying the clinical tests used to diagnose this disorder.

Introduction

The hypothalamus and pituitary gland are the principal organizers of the endocrine system. The hypothalamus is part of the brain and is directly connected to the pituitary gland. The hypothalamus receives a wide range of neural inputs that can alter its secretory functions in response to conditions such as stress, exercise and even the time of day. It is subject to negative feedback regulation by both pituitary and target organ hormones. Because of this complex set of inputs and outputs, the hypothalamus acts to integrate many hormonal and neural responses (Fig. 2.1).

The pituitary has two quite distinct parts: the posterior pituitary, which is an extension of nerve cells from the hypothalamus, and the anterior pituitary, which is linked by blood vessels from the hypothalamus. The hypothalamus controls the function of both the anterior and posterior pituitary, but achieves this in different ways. The hormones secreted by the posterior pituitary are synthesized in nerve cells in the hypothalamus and transported along nerve axons to the posterior pituitary, from which they are simply released from the nerve terminals. However, the hypothalamus also produces a range of hormones that act on the different cell types of the anterior pituitary to control their secretory activity. These releasing and inhibitory hormones travel from the hypothalamus to the anterior pituitary in a network of blood vessels called a portal circulation.

One of the main functions of the anterior pituitary is to secrete hormones that control the activity of other endocrine glands, particularly the gonads, thyroid and adrenal. So it can be seen that the hypothalamus and pituitary are the master controllers of several completely independent endocrine systems, such as the hypothalamo–pituitary–adrenal axis (HPA axis) and the hypothalamo–pituitary–gonadal axis.

Interesting fact

The parts of the pituitary gland have been called by different names at different times: posterior pituitary = neurohypophysis; anterior pituitary = adenohypophysis.

The word 'pituitary' derives from the wonderfully onomatopoeic Greek word *ptuo* (to spit), hence the Latin *pituita* (mucus). This is because it was once thought that the function of the pituitary was to allow mucus produced by the brain to drain down the nose!

Hypothalamic tumour box 1

Case history

Mr Jones, a 30-year-old man, began passing a lot of urine approximately 6 weeks earlier. He needed to pass urine once or twice per hour and was woken from his sleep by a full bladder at least four or five times. He felt unusually thirsty, was constantly drinking water and had noticed that his urine was very pale. In recent weeks he had been having headaches at night and on waking. His libido had decreased over recent months and he had problems maintaining an erection. Most recently he had become very forgetful.

The medical history was unremarkable. Mr Jones lived with his girlfriend and they had no children. He worked as an engineer.

He had been to see his GP, who had tested his urine and found no protein or glucose present. The GP also found no abnormalities in Mr Jones' blood glucose or calcium levels. At this stage the GP referred Mr Jones to an endocrine clinic.

On examination in the clinic he looked uncomfortable and dehydrated with a dry mouth and tongue. His temperature was normal, 37°C, but the resting pulse rate was 100 beats per minute, with a blood pressure of 105/65 mmHg. Fundoscopy revealed the optic nerve to be swollen in both eyes. Testing of the visual fields showed a loss of vision in both temporal (outer) halves of the field (see Fig. 2.3). He was confused and could not remember how he had got to the hospital or what he had eaten that day, but he knew the name of his girlfriend and could remember distant events.

Where can I find the hypothalamus and pituitary?

As its name implies, the hypothalamus is located beneath the thalamus at the base of the brain. The hypothalamus is closely related to the optic chiasm (inferiorly), mamillary bodies (posteriorly) and the third ventricle (superiorly) (Fig. 2.2).

The hypothalamus is a part of the brain that acts as a control centre for a range of diverse processes, including regulation of the autonomic nervous system, body temperature, water balance, appetite and mood. It does this by integrating monitoring processes with regulatory systems, and neural processes with endocrine systems. For example, the hypothalamus contains cells that produce the anti-diuretic hormone,

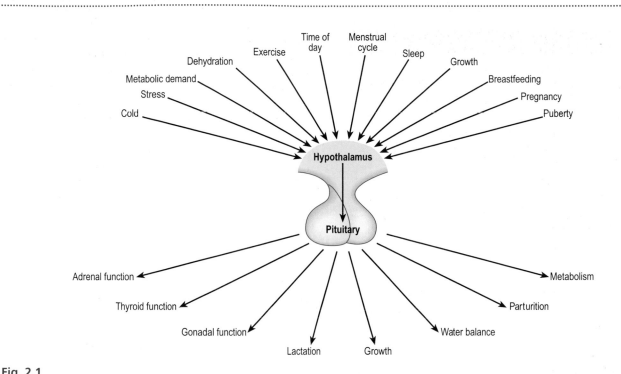

Fig. 2.1
Integrative functions of the hypothalamus and pituitary. Both external and internal cues are relayed through the hypothalamus, leading to hormone secretion from the pituitary. The pituitary hormones regulate a number of important physiological processes.

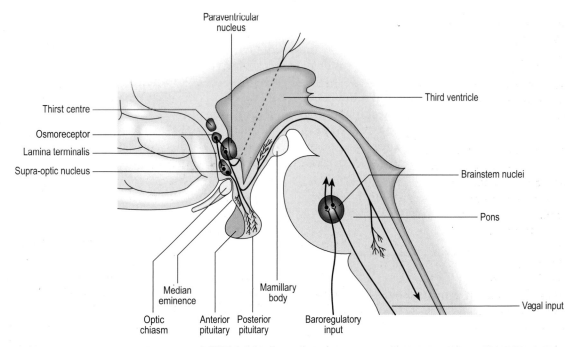

Fig. 2.2
Diagram of the location of the hypothalamus and pituitary.

arginine vasopressin, cells that monitor the concentration of plasma (osmoreceptors), and an area that regulates thirst, all connected by a neural network. The areas of the hypothalamus that are anatomically or functionally distinct are known as nuclei. Several of the hypothalamic nuclei have primarily endocrine functions, most notably the paraventricular nucleus, but also the supra-optic and ventromedial nuclei.

THE HYPOTHALAMUS AND POSTERIOR PITUITARY

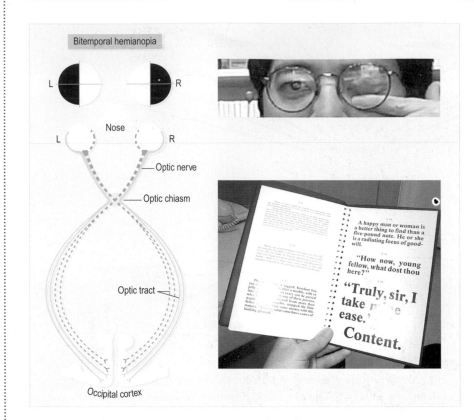

Fig. 2.3
This picture shows the type of visual disturbance that may occur when a pituitary tumour compresses the optic chiasm. This is called a bilateral hemianopia. The dotted line indicates the visual pathways affected: the light falling on the nasal side of the retina is not detected. Visual fields are assessed by the ability to see a coloured object as it is moved through the visual field. Visual acuity is assessed with a J chart. (Reproduced from Chew S L, Leslie D 2006 Clinical endocrinology and diabetes: an illustrated colour text. Churchill Livingstone, Edinburgh.)

These are located in the region of the hypothalamus close to the third ventricle.

The hypothalamus is physically connected to the pituitary gland by the pituitary stalk. The pituitary gland is located in the pituitary fossa, which is a hollow in the sphenoid bone at the base of the brain (see Fig. 2.2). The pituitary lies outside the blood–brain barrier and is not considered to be a part of the brain. Anatomically the pituitary gland is very close to the optic chiasm and large pituitary tumours often cause visual disturbances (Fig. 2.3). The normal pituitary gland weighs less than 1g and is approximately 14mm across, although it increases in size during pregnancy and shrinks with age.

> **Interesting fact**
>
> The pituitary fossa is also known as the sella turcica, due to its apparent resemblance to a Turkish style of saddle. More bizarrely, 'hypothalamus' comes from the Greek for 'under the bed'!

Connection between the hypothalamus and pituitary

The pituitary stalk, which connects the hypothalamus to the pituitary gland, carries both blood vessels and nerve fibres. The anterior pituitary is connected to the hypothalamus by a vascular connection through the hypophyseal portal system. A portal system is a vascular connection with two sets of capillary beds. The first set of capillaries is in the hypothalamus and blood passes through the portal veins in the pituitary stalk to the second set of capillaries in the anterior pituitary (Fig. 2.4). In this way, agents released from the hypothalamus can be delivered to the pituitary where they act on pituitary cells to control hormone synthesis and release.

The posterior pituitary consists of fibres of the magnocellular and parvocellular neurons, which carry the posterior pituitary hormones from the hypothalamus.

Development of the hypothalamus and pituitary

The posterior pituitary is neural in origin and, together with the pituitary stalk, derives from a down-growth of the diencephalon. The anterior pituitary is ectodermal and derives from Rathke's pouch, an outgrowth of the buccal cavity. The two tissues migrate to lie adjacent to each other and form the pituitary gland. The anterior component is larger than the posterior part, comprising about two-thirds of the gland.

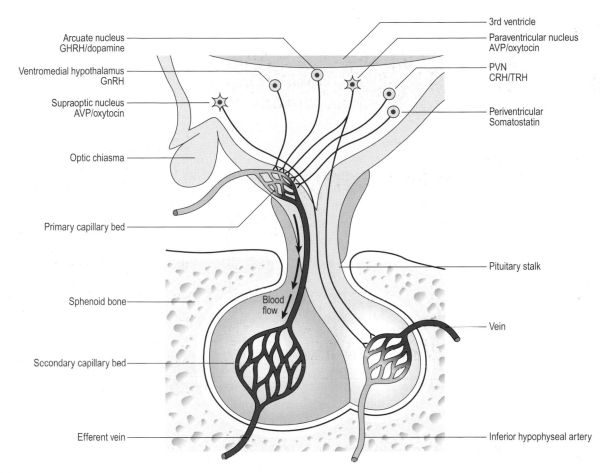

Fig. 2.4
Neural and vascular connections between the hypothalamus and pituitary. The hypothalamus and posterior pituitary have a direct neural link, whereas the anterior pituitary has a vascular connection to the hypothalamus. Note the separate blood supply to the two parts of the pituitary. Disruption of the portal system results in failure of anterior pituitary hormone secretion, but usually not of posterior pituitary hormones. The neurons with star-shaped cell bodies are magnocellular neurons and the round cell bodies indicate parvocellular neurons. AVP, arginine vasopressin; CRH, corticotropin releasing hormone; GnRH, gonadotropin releasing hormone; PVN, paraventricular nucleus; TRH, thyrotropin releasing hormone.

Hypothalamic tumour box 2

Case note: Investigation

Given the combination of abnormal regulation of water balance and visual disturbance, can you localize the problem area?

The main site of control of water excretion is the hypothalamus, which contains both osmoreceptors and cells that produce the anti-diuretic hormone, vasopressin. A homonymous bitemporal hemianopia is characteristic of lesions of the optic chiasm. So the combination of these two features would suggest a lesion affecting both the hypothalamus and the optic chiasm.

What further tests would you want to carry out?

Blood and urine tests were performed and showed serum levels of sodium 154 mmol/L, serum urea 15 mmol/L, plasma glucose 8.2 mmol/L, and urine osmolality <50 mOsm/kg and serum osmolality >295 mOsm/kg.

An MRI scan was performed and showed a large tumour of the hypothalamus with pressure or infiltration of the surrounding structures (Fig. 2.5).

Psychometric testing by a psychologist would be helpful as a baseline to quantify the extent of Mr Jones' short-term memory problem.

THE HYPOTHALAMUS AND POSTERIOR PITUITARY

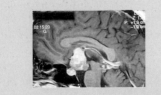

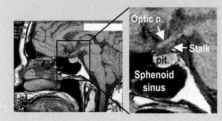

Fig. 2.5
Magnetic resonance images of the pituitary gland and hypothalamus in the sagittal plane. The top image shows the tumour destroying Mr. Jones' hypothalamus. The irregular tumour contains many blood vessels and shows a bright signal after contrast injection. The lower image shows a normal pituitary and hypothalamic anatomy.

The hormones of the posterior pituitary

The posterior pituitary secretes two hormones, oxytocin and vasopressin. Vasopressin is also called arginine vasopressin (AVP) or sometimes anti-diuretic hormone (ADH) because of its major physiological action. Both oxytocin and arginine vasopressin are small peptides, of only nine amino acids, seven of which are common to both (Fig. 2.6). They are synthesized in the hypothalamus, in the magnocellular neurons of the supra-optic and paraventricular nuclei (see Fig. 2.4). Different subsets of the neurons produce either oxytocin or arginine vasopressin. They are both made as part of a large precursor peptide called neurophysin, which is processed into the mature peptide hormones as it passes along the neural tract. These hormones are transported down the nerve axons in the supra-optic–hypothalamic tract into the posterior pituitary. Release of oxytocin or arginine vasopressin is brought about by an action potential in the nerve.

Arginine vasopressin

$$\text{Cys} - \text{Tyr} - \text{Phe} - \text{Gln} - \text{Asn} - \text{Cys} - \text{Pro} - \text{Arg} - \text{Gly} - \text{NH}_2$$

Oxytocin

$$\text{Cys} - \text{Tyr} - \text{Ile} - \text{Gln} - \text{Asn} - \text{Cys} - \text{Pro} - \text{Leu} - \text{Gly} - \text{NH}_2$$

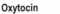

Fig. 2.6
Structures of oxytocin and vasopressin.

Release of posterior pituitary hormones is part of a neuroendocrine reflex: oxytocin secretion and actions

A neuroendocrine reflex involves the release of a hormone from a nerve terminal in response to depolarization of the nerve (Fig. 2.7). It differs from simple

① Baby suckling

② Sensory nerve activation

③ Activation of magnocellular neurons

④ Action potential to posterior pituitary

⑤ Release of oxytocin into blood

⑥ Acts on smooth muscle in milk ducts to expel milk

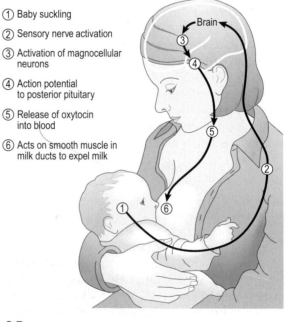

Fig. 2.7
Neuroendocrine reflex. Suckling of the baby causes a sensory nerve signal to be sent to the brain. The signal is relayed to the hypothalamus where activation of magnocellular neurons causes release of the hormone oxytocin from the posterior pituitary. Oxytocin travels in blood and acts on the primed breast ducts, causing smooth muscle contraction and milk expulsion.

neurotransmission because the hormone is released into blood, rather than a synaptic cleft. The control of oxytocin release makes a good illustration of the principles of a neuroendocrine reflex. This hormone has a role in both parturition (childbirth) and lactation. It does not influence the production of milk, but is essential for the release of milk: the milk ejection reflex. During lactation, suckling initiates a neural signal from the nipple to the brain. This signal is relayed to the hypothalamus and an action potential is sent along the neural tract to the posterior pituitary, causing the release of oxytocin from the posterior pituitary into the bloodstream. The oxytocin acts on the smooth muscle surrounding the alveoli in the breast, causing contraction of the muscle and ejection of milk from the nipple.

The role of oxytocin in men is unclear and in women its role is clearly limited to very specific situations. Therapeutically, oxytocin is used to increase uterine contractions and to reduce postpartum bleeding.

Regulation of vasopressin secretion

Like oxytocin, arginine vasopressin release is part of a neuroendocrine reflex. The major stimulus to the release of arginine vasopressin is an increase in plasma osmolality (Box 2.1), which is detected by osmoreceptors in the hypothalamus (Fig. 2.8). A neural signal is relayed to the paraventricular and supra-optic nuclei and an action potential is generated in the nerves supplying the posterior pituitary, causing the release of arginine vasopressin into the blood. A decrease in either blood volume or blood pressure also stimulates the release of arginine vasopressin. A fall in blood volume is detected by the baroreceptors in the left atrium of the heart, whereas a decreased blood pressure is detected by the baroreceptors in the aortic arch and carotid artery. However, the most important factor in regulating arginine vasopressin secretion is plasma osmolality, with a normal threshold of 280 mmol/kg. This threshold is slightly lower in pregnancy and significantly reduced by a fall in blood volume.

Actions of arginine vasopressin
(Table 2.1)

Arginine vasopressin is a short-acting hormone, with a plasma half-life of around 15 minutes. Its main site of action is the collecting duct of the kidney, where it increases water resorption by making the ducts more permeable to water (see Fig. 2.8). It achieves this by

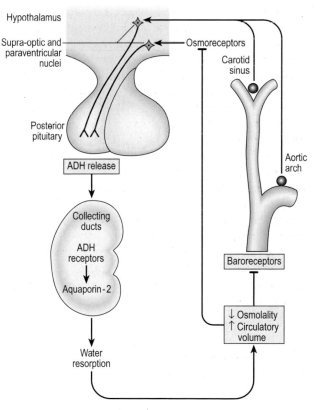

Fig. 2.8
Regulation and action of vasopressin (ADH, anti-diuretic hormone). This is another example of a neuroendocrine reflex: the baroreceptors in the aortic arch and carotid sinus send neural signals to the hypothalamus, resulting in the release of a hormone, ADH. (Reproduced from Chew S L, Leslie D 2006 Clinical endocrinology and diabetes: an illustrated colour text. Churchill Livingstone, Edinburgh.)

Box 2.1

What is plasma osmolality?

The amount of osmotically active particles in a biological fluid is expressed in osmoles. Technically, the osmolality is the number of osmoles per kilogram of solvent (plasma or urine) and is the primary measure of concentration. The very similar term 'osmolarity' refers to the number of osmoles per *litre* of solvent. As 1 litre of water weighs 1 kg, these two terms tend to be used interchangeably. More than 90% of the solute in plasma is sodium and its associated anions, chloride and bicarbonate. Glucose and urea make up most of the remaining solutes. The concentration of solute determines the freezing point of a liquid and this is how osmolality is measured in the laboratory. The osmolality of plasma can also be estimated by the formula:

Osmolality (mOsm/L) = 2 × sodium (mmol/L) + glucose (mmol/L) + urea (mmol/L).

Table 2.1
Actions of arginine vasopressin (anti-diuretic hormone)

Tissue	Receptor subtype	Effect
Kidney	V_2 receptor	Anti-diuresis (by increasing water reabsorption)
Pituitary gland (corticotroph cells)	V_{1b} receptor	Stimulates release of ACTH (acts with CRH)
Vascular smooth muscle	V_{1a} receptor	Causes vasoconstriction
Vascular endothelial cells	V_2 receptor	Release of clotting factors

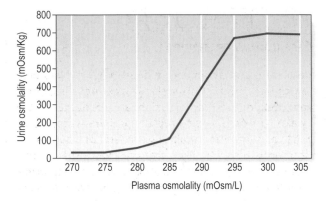

Fig. 2.9
Effects of vasopressin on the kidney: the relationship between plasma and urine osmolalities. As plasma osmolality increases, the actions of AVP (ADH) cause an increase in urine osmolality until a plateau is reached. (From Chew S L, Leslie D 2006 Clinical endocrinology and diabetes: an illustrated colour text. Churchill Livingstone, Edinburgh.)

binding to the V_2 subclass of receptors on the basolateral surface of cells lining the renal collecting ducts. The effect of activating these vasopressin receptors is to stimulate production of a protein called aquaporin 2 on the apical membrane of these cells. Aquaporin 2 forms an open channel that allows water to pass out of the lumen of the collecting duct. The physiological effect of arginine vasopressin is the conservation of water in the body by causing the production of smaller volumes of more highly concentrated urine, which may be more than twice the osmolality of plasma (Fig. 2.9). As its name implies, arginine vasopressin also has actions on the vascular system, causing increases in blood pressure through the activation of vasopressin V_1 receptors in blood vessels. The vasopressin receptors in the kidney (called V_2) are slightly different from those in blood vessels (called V_1).

This is exploited in the development of drugs that bind preferentially to V_2 receptors and so can be used to treat diabetes insipidus without adverse effects on blood pressure.

Interesting fact

Most peptide hormones have to be administered by injection. However, desmopressin, the synthetic analogue of arginine vasopressin, can be administered orally in tablet form, or by nasal spray. However, there is a difference in the dose required depending on the route of administration: given orally the effective dose is 100 µg, by nasal spray it is 10–20 µg, but when administered by subcutaneous injection only 1 µg is required.

Hypothalamic tumour box 3

Case note: Explanation of symptoms and signs

When vasopressin secretion is damaged, as in Mr Jones' case, aquaporin 2 no longer forms a water channel for reabsorption of water, and water loss in the urine results in large volumes of dilute urine. Thirst and excessive drinking are caused by a high concentration of plasma, due to water losses in the urine. This condition is called diabetes insipidus. The consequent dehydration results in decreased blood volume with increased pulse rate and hypotension.

The visual impairment is due to compression of the optic chiasm, resulting in optic neuritis and homonymous bitemporal hemianopia. The loss of short-term memory is due to damage to the mamillary bodies. Both of these effects are due to space-occupying effects of the tumour on adjacent structures.

The headaches on waking are a classical symptom of an intra-cranial mass, which causes stretching of the dura mater.

Impaired sexual function can result from any disease of the pituitary or hypothalamus that impairs gonadotropin production.

Disorders of vasopressin secretion and action

Deficiency

A deficiency of arginine vasopressin secretion or action results in a condition termed diabetes insipidus. Diabetes insipidus is called 'hypothalamic' or 'cranial' when there is a failure of arginine vasopressin secretion, and 'nephrogenic' when there is renal insensitivity to the actions of arginine vasopressin ('vasopressin resistance'). The two conditions are easily distinguished by giving the patient desmopressin and testing the response of urine concentration. In cranial diabetes insipidus, the urine becomes very concentrated (i.e. the urine volume drops and urine osmolality rises). Conversely, in nephrogenic diabetes insipidus, the urine does not change in response to desmopressin administration.

Diabetes insipidus is characterized by polyuria, the production of large volumes of very dilute urine, accompanied by polydipsia, excessive thirst. There is no single cause of either hypothalamic or nephrogenic diabetes insipidus: neither is a common disorder. However, the hypothalamic form may be caused by a tumour, or may result from trauma to the brain. It may be caused by surgery to adjacent areas, such as the pituitary gland, and in these cases the disorder is often transient. Hypothalamic diabetes insipidus is treated by administration of a synthetic analogue of vasopressin, termed desmopressin, which has all the renal effects of vasopressin but has less effect on the vasculature because of much weaker binding to V_1 vasopressin receptors.

Nephrogenic diabetes insipidus occasionally results from a genetic defect in vasopressin receptors, although this is rare. More commonly it is a result of metabolic disturbances, such as hypercalcaemia, or seen as an adverse drug reaction. It is a recognized complication of lithium therapy, which is used to treat bipolar disorder. Nephrogenic diabetes insipidus is usually treated by correcting the underlying metabolic problem or discontinuing drug therapy. However, it may also be treated with drugs that increase renal sensitivity to arginine vasopressin, such as chlorpropamide.

Other causes of polyuria, polydipsia and thirst include diabetes mellitus (distinguished by abnormally high blood sugar levels) and primary polydipsia. There are several causes of primary polydipsia, including psychogenic (where patients with mental illness drink tens of litres of water per day) and idiopathic (where otherwise healthy people have a lowered osmotic threshold for thirst). Primary polydipsia can usually be distinguished from diabetes insipidus by the fact that the plasma is dilute, rather than concentrated. A water deprivation test may also be useful: in primary polydipsia the urine becomes appropriately concentrated on dehydration; in hypothalamic diabetes insipidus the urine becomes appropriately concentrated only after desmopressin is given, and in nephrogenic diabetes insipidus the urine osmolality does not change with either dehydration or desmopressin.

Interesting fact

Before the advent of modern methods of urine analysis, the only way to test urine was for the physician to dip their finger into a sample and taste it. This is how the two types of diabetes got their names: in diabetes mellitus (a disorder of glucose metabolism) the urine characteristically tastes sweet, whereas in diabetes insipidus (a disorder of water metabolism) the urine was considered to 'lack flavour'.

Hypothalamic tumour box 4

Case note: Management

How can treatment be guided by physiological principles? The first principle of treatment is to prevent dehydration by ensuring an adequate water intake. The second is to replace arginine vasopressin with a synthetic analogue called desmopressin. Desmopressin acts like arginine vasopressin and reduces urinary water excretion and increases urine osmolality. Finally, the underlying disease process must be treated, by surgical removal of the tumour, although destruction of the hypothalamic nuclei may leave permanent diabetes insipidus. The damage that has been caused to adjacent structures is also likely to be irreversible, leaving Mr Jones with permanent disability.

Excess arginine vasopressin secretion

Excess vasopressin secretion results in the syndrome of inappropriate anti-diuretic hormone (SIADH) where the water retention has such a diluting effect on plasma that it results in low plasma sodium levels (hyponatraemia) with a normal plasma volume. SIADH has many causes including neoplasms such as lung cancer, neurological disorders such as meningitis, lung disease such as pneumonia, and prescribed drugs such as carbamazepine.

Thirst

If you look at Figure 2.1, the connection between dehydration acting on the hypothalamus and, as a result, the pituitary acting to regulate water balance, is thirst. Thirst is such a common experience that we assume it is a simple process, but the regulation of thirst is very complex, involving angiotensin II, arginine vasopressin, and central and peripheral receptors.

Water intoxication occurs when an individual drinks more fluids than they can handle in a physiologically appropriate manner. It can have many causes, including the psychogenic polydipsia associated with schizophrenia, and the excessive drinking seen following ingestion of Ecstasy (MDMA), which usually occurs in a misguided attempt to avoid dehydration and hyperthermia.

Hypothalamic tumour box 5

A suggested exercise

Estimate Mr Jones' plasma osmolality: sodium concentration 154 mmol/L, urea 15 mmol/L and glucose 8 mmol/L.

(Answer: $[2 \times 154] + 15 + 8 = 331$ mOsm/L)

The osmolality of Mr Jones' urine was <50 mOsm/kg. What would it be if he did not have diabetes insipidus and his serum osmolality was 331 mOsm/L?

(Answer: It should be greater than $2 \times 331 = 662$ mOsm/kg)

Extended matching questions

A   Anterior pituitary
B   Aortic arch
C   Collecting ducts of the kidney
D   Hypothalamo–pituitary portal system
E   Hypothalamus
F   Juxta-glomerular apparatus of the kidney
G   Magnocellular neurons
H   Optic chiasm
I   Parvocellular neurons
J   Posterior pituitary
K   Right atrium
L   Vascular smooth muscle cells throughout the body

For each of the descriptions below select the anatomical location from the list above that best matches the description:

① The route by which arginine vasopressin (AVP) gets from its site of synthesis to its site of release.

② The location of AVP V_2 receptors.

③ The site of baroreceptors that respond to a fall in blood pressure.

④ The site where AVP acts as a releasing hormone.

⑤ The site of chemoreceptors that are responsive to a rise in plasma osmolality.

⑥ The site of release of oxytocin.

Answers see page 150

THE HYPOTHALAMUS AND PITUITARY PART II: THE ANTERIOR PITUITARY

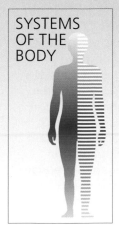

SYSTEMS OF THE BODY

Chapter objectives

After reading this chapter you should be able to:

① Describe the structure of the anterior pituitary and the hormones produced by each cell type.

② Describe how the secretion of each anterior pituitary hormone is regulated.

③ Describe the physiological effects of each anterior pituitary hormone.

④ Describe the effects of under- and over-production of growth hormone.

⑤ Describe the regulation and actions of prolactin.

⑥ Explain the science underlying the clinical tests used to diagnose disorders of growth hormone secretion.

Acromegaly box 1

Case history 1

Mr Roberts, a 65-year-old man, was admitted to hospital for a routine repair of a hernia. The anaesthetist who assessed him before the operation noticed that he had a very large jaw and tongue. The anaesthetist was concerned about the difficulty of maintaining the airway during the operation and so the operation was postponed and an endocrinologist was called.

Why do you think that the anaesthetist called for an endocrine opinion on Mr Roberts? The answer is that the anaesthetist was fairly sure that Mr Roberts had a hormonal disorder called acromegaly (from the Greek *acro*, meaning extremity, and *megaly*, meaning great). Acromegaly is caused by excessive secretion of growth hormone and classically results in growth of soft tissues and peripheries (hands, feet and face). Nearly all cases are due to a benign adenoma of the anterior pituitary.

Just as in Mr Roberts' case, acromegaly is a classical 'foot of the bed' diagnosis. In other words, you can make the diagnosis simply from the characteristic appearance of the patient (Fig. 3.1).

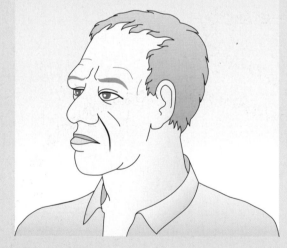

Fig. 3.1
Mr Roberts' face shows some typical features of acromegaly: skin growth has resulted in coarsening of his features, with exaggeration of the eyebrow ridge and skin folds on his face. His jaw is enlarged and his skin has become rather greasy.

The hormones of the anterior pituitary

The anterior pituitary is composed of five different cell types, each of which secretes a different hormone (Table 3.1). These hormones are all peptides (Fig. 3.2).

Table 3.1
Major cell types of the anterior pituitary and the hormones they secrete

Cell type	Hormone	Structure	Size
Acidophil cells			
Somatotrophs	Growth hormone	Protein	~22 000 Da 191 amino acids
Lactotrophs	Prolactin	Protein	~23 000 Da 198 amino acids
Basophil cells			
Thyrotrophs	TSH	Glycoprotein	~30 000 Da
Gonadotrophs	LH and FSH	Glycoproteins	~25 000 Da
Corticotrophs	ACTH	Peptide	39 amino acids

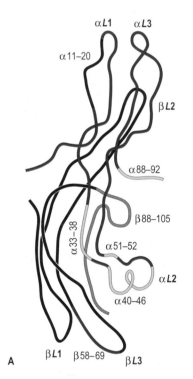

Fig. 3.2
Structures of anterior pituitary hormones. (A) TSH is a large peptide hormone consisting of two polypeptide chains. This diagram shows the tertiary structure of TSH. The α chain is shown as a grey line and the β chain as a black line. The folding of the peptides, producing the hairpin loops, is essential for the hormone's biological activity. The loops are labelled αL1–3 on the α chain, and βL1–3 on the β chain. Other biologically important areas of the hormone are indicated. For clarity, the carbohydrate chains which are attached to the peptide have not been illustrated. The gonadotropins, LH and FSH, have a similar structure. (Redrawn from Physiological Review 2002; 82: 473–502, with permission).

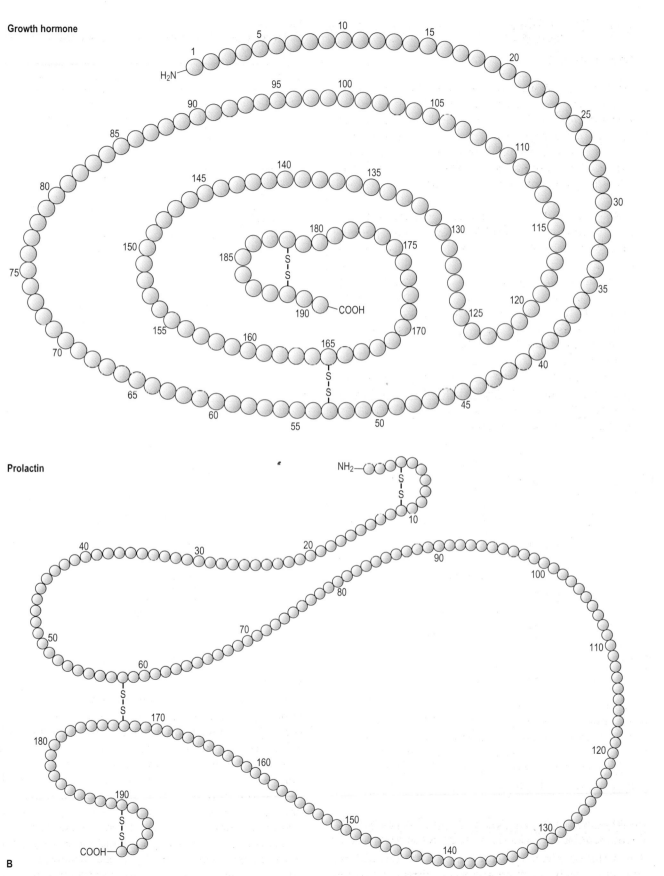

Growth hormone

Prolactin

Fig. 3.2 (Continued)
(B) Growth hormone and prolactin. These are large, single-chain peptide hormones with disulphide bridges important in maintaining the tertiary structure of the hormones.

27

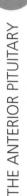
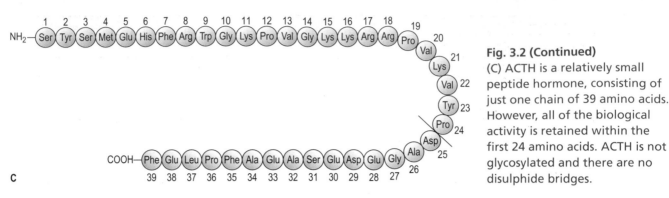

Fig. 3.2 (Continued)
(C) ACTH is a relatively small peptide hormone, consisting of just one chain of 39 amino acids. However, all of the biological activity is retained within the first 24 amino acids. ACTH is not glycosylated and there are no disulphide bridges.

Pro-opiomelanocortin

N-terminal peptide fragment 1–131	ACTH 1–39	β-Lipotrophin 1–91

β-endorphin
Met-enkephalin
γ-Melanocyte stimulating hormone

Fig. 3.3

Pro-opiomelanocortin is a large precursor peptide that gives rise to a number of biologically active peptides, including β-endorphin, involved in the endogenous control of pain, and ACTH, the major regulator of adrenal function. The N-terminal fragment is thought to have a role in stimulating adrenal growth.

Prolactin and growth hormone are large single-chain polypeptides that have considerable sequence homology. Luteinizing hormone (LH), follicle stimulating hormone (FSH) and thyroid stimulating hormone (TSH) are members of a family of large double-chained glycoproteins that includes human chorionic gonadotropin (hCG). These hormones consist of two glycosylated polypeptide chains linked by disulphide bridges. The α subunit is identical for all members of this hormone family and it is the hormone-specific β subunit that distinguishes these hormones. Adrenocorticotropic hormone (ACTH) is relatively small, comprising just 39 amino acids, but it is synthesized as part of a much larger precursor protein, termed pro-opiomelanocortin (POMC), which also gives rise to β-endorphin and the opioid peptides met- and leu-enkephalin (Fig. 3.3).

Regulation of hormone secretion in the anterior pituitary

The secretion of each of the anterior pituitary peptides is under a complex control system, involving both negative feedback and hypothalamic regulation by factors released from the hypothalamus into the portal system supplying the anterior pituitary. Most

Table 3.2
Major hypothalamic factors and their actions

Hormone	Acronym	Structure (no. of amino acids)	Action
Thyrotropin releasing hormone	TRH	3	↑ TSH release
Gonadotropin releasing hormone	GnRH	10	↑ LH and FSH release
Corticotropin releasing hormone	CRH	44	↑ ACTH release
Arginine vasopressin	AVP	9	↑ ACTH release
Growth hormone releasing hormone	GHRH	44	↑ GH release
Somatostatin		14	↓GH release
Dopamine	Catecholamine		↓ Prolactin release

of the anterior pituitary hormones are regulated by 'stimulating factors' from the hypothalamus, but both growth hormone and prolactin are also regulated by hypothalamic 'release-inhibiting factors'. Most of the hypothalamic releasing and release-inhibiting factors are peptide hormones (Table 3.2 and Fig. 3.4), but some neurotransmitters, such as dopamine, are also involved. When considering the anterior pituitary, the four 'tropic hormones' are often considered separately. The tropic hormones are those hormones that regulate other endocrine glands: LH, FSH, ACTH and TSH. The regulation of these hormones will be considered in more detail in Chapters 4–7. For the remainder of this chapter we will focus on prolactin and growth hormone.

Acromegaly box 2

Case history 2

The full history revealed that Mr Roberts had slowly and insidiously developed swelling of the hands and feet over about 5 years. He was no longer able

Hormone	Structure
Thyrotropin releasing hormone (TRH)	(pyro)Glu–His–Pro–NH$_2$
Gonadotropin releasing hormone (GnRH)	(pyro)Glu–His–Trp–Ser–Tyr–Gly–Leu–Arg–Pro–Gly–NH$_2$
Somatostatin	Ala–Gly–Cys–Lys–Asn–Phe–Phe–Trp–Lys–Thr–Phe–Thr–Ser–Cys (with S–S bridges)
Growth hormone releasing hormone (GHRH)	Tyr–Ala–Asp–Ala–Ile–Phe–Thr–Asn–Ser–Tyr–Arg–Lys–Val–Leu–Gly–Gln–Leu–Ser–Ala–Arg–Lys–Leu–Leu–Gln–Asp–Ile–Met–Ser–Arg–Gln–Gln–Gly–Glu–Ser–Asn–Gln–Glu–Arg–Gly–Ala–Arg–Ala–Arg–Leu–NH$_2$
Dopamine (inhibits prolactin secretion)	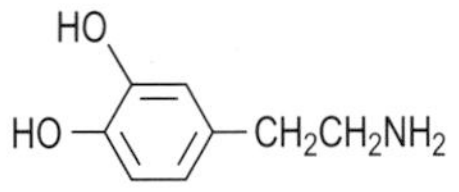 HO–(ring)(HO)–CH$_2$CH$_2$NH$_2$
Corticotropin releasing hormone (CRH)	Ser–Gln–Glu–Pro–Pro–Ile–Ser–Leu–Asp–Leu–Thr–Phe–His–Leu–Leu–Arg–Glu–Val–Leu–Glu–Met–Thr–Lys–Ala–Asp–Gln–Leu–Ala–Gln–Gln–Ala–His–Ser–Asn–Arg–Lys–Leu–Leu–Asp–Ile–Ala–NH$_2$
Arginine vasopressin	Cys–Tyr–Phe–Gln–Asn–Cys–Pro–Arg–Gly–NH$_2$ (with S–S bridge)

Fig. 3.4
Structures of hypothalamic hormones involved in regulating anterior pituitary function.

to wear his wedding ring and had had to buy larger shoes. He complained of pins and needles in his hands and increased sweating, both particularly at night. In the last few years he had noted pain in the left hip on walking.

On examination, Mr Roberts had large hands and feet with thick doughy palms. His jaw was large and the lower teeth protruded in front of the upper teeth (Fig. 3.5). His tongue was large and his teeth were widely separated. His chest was large and shaped like a barrel and his blood pressure was 155/95 mmHg.

The blood tests showed a plasma glucose level of 12 mmol/L, but normal electrolytes, renal and liver function, and blood count.

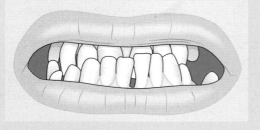

Fig. 3.5
In acromegaly, the excess growth hormone causes the lower mandible, a flat bone, to grow. This causes the lower teeth to protrude beyond the upper teeth. Acromegaly may initially be noticed by the dentist, when a patient's teeth change or dentures no longer fit.

Regulation of growth hormone secretion (Fig. 3.6)
The hypothalamus secretes two peptides that exert opposing effects and together regulate growth hormone secretion. Growth hormone releasing hormone stimulates growth hormone release, whereas somatostatin exerts an inhibitory effect. It is the balance between these two hormones that determines the rate of growth hormone secretion. The major physiological stimulus for growth hormone secretion is the onset of sleep. In both adults and children there is a marked diurnal variation in growth hormone secretion with a peak occurring 1–2 hours after the onset of sleep (Fig. 3.7). The secretion of growth hormone is also stimulated by stress, exercise, the presence of certain amino acids in plasma (especially arginine) and by a fall in plasma glucose concentrations. It is suppressed by high plasma glucose levels. These effects can be used therapeutically to investigate disorders of growth hormone secretion.

There is also a negative feedback component in the regulation of growth hormone secretion, both by growth hormone itself and by insulin-like growth factor 1 (IGF-1) (see below, Actions of growth hormone). These feedback effects are on both the hypothalamus and the pituitary.

Regulation of prolactin secretion
Prolactin is unique among the major hormones in that its secretion is mainly under inhibitory control. Experimentally, several hormones have been shown to stimulate prolactin release, and for a long time there was a search for the 'prolactin releasing factor'. It is now clear, however, that prolactin secretion is under

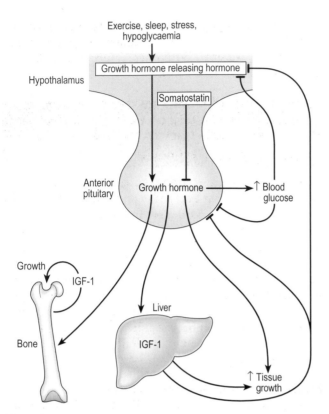

Fig. 3.6

The regulation of growth hormone (GH) secretion. Two hypothalamic hormones regulate GH secretion: growth hormone releasing hormone and somatostatin. The balance between these hormones determines the rate of GH secretion. GH exerts many of its effects indirectly, through the production and action of IGF-1.

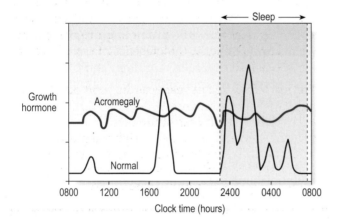

Fig. 3.7

Diurnal pattern of GH secretion. During the day GH levels are often too low to measure. Secretion of GH increases during periods of sleep, particularly at the start of sleep, and there are also 'spikes' of secretion during the day. The secretion of GH is described as 'episodic'. In acromegaly there is less variation in GH levels throughout the day and the level of GH never becomes undetectable. The plasma half-life of GH is about 30 minutes.

Acromegaly box 3

Case note: Establishing the diagnosis

Measurement of serum growth hormone

Normally growth hormone secretion is controlled by a negative feedback loop involving IGF-1. However, in acromegaly the pituitary adenoma secretes growth hormone in a manner that is relatively resistant to feedback regulation. In addition to higher levels of growth hormone, the pattern of secretion is altered. Normally, growth hormone is secreted at night and is often undetectable during the day, whereas in acromegaly pulses of growth hormone are made throughout the night and day, the diurnal rhythm is lost, and growth hormone is never undetectable (see Fig. 3.7). To confirm the diagnosis, growth hormone will be found in detectable amounts during the day and serum IGF-1 levels will be high.

Oral glucose test (Fig. 3.8).

This is very similar to the test used to confirm diabetes mellitus. A fixed dose of glucose is given orally after an overnight fast and serum hormone levels are measured at intervals. Oral glucose normally suppresses growth hormone to undetectable levels, but in acromegaly the levels are not suppressible.

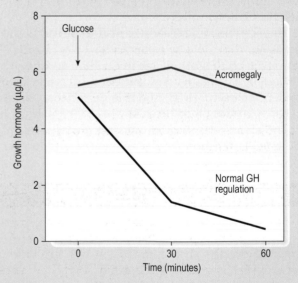

Fig. 3.8

Glucose suppression of GH secretion. An oral dose of glucose is given after a period of fasting. Blood GH levels are measured at 0, 30 and 60 minutes after the glucose load. In a normal person, the level of GH should be lower than 2 µg/L at 30 and 60 minutes. In a person with acromegaly the GH is not suppressed and may even show a paradoxical increase.

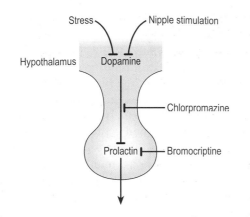

Fig. 3.9
Regulation of prolactin secretion. Prolactin is under *tonic inhibitory control* by dopamine. This means that prolactin is released only when dopamine secretion by the hypothalamus is inhibited. Drugs that mimic dopamine, such as bromocriptine, inhibit prolactin, but dopamine *antagonists*, such as chlorpromazine, stimulate prolactin release. There does not appear to be any negative feedback regulation in the control of prolactin secretion.

tonic inhibitory control, principally by dopamine released from the hypothalamus. If the inhibitory effect of dopamine is removed then secretion of prolactin occurs (Fig. 3.9). There remains a possibility that other minor factors are involved in both inhibiting and stimulating prolactin secretion.

The major physiological stimulus to prolactin secretion is suckling. Prolactin levels also rise during the latter half of pregnancy, an effect that is thought to be mediated by oestradiol. Prolactin secretion is also increased during sleep and by stress and exercise. There is a short negative feedback loop involving prolactin itself causing an increase in hypothalamic dopamine levels.

Stress hormones

Several of the anterior pituitary hormones are known as 'stress hormones' as their secretion increases in response to stress. These include ACTH, growth hormone, prolactin and to some extent TSH. The 'stress' can be either physical, such as exercise, or psychological, such as exam stress. Paradigms exist for testing different forms of stress under laboratory conditions; the standard psychological stressor is performing mental arithmetic in front of an audience. Standard physiological stressors include the cold stressor test which involves plunging your arm into a bucket of ice water for a fixed period of time. Other stressors that stimulate the secretion of these hormones include exercise, hypoglycaemia induced by insulin administration (see

section below on hypopituitarism), sleep deprivation, infection and pyrexia. Non-pituitary stress hormones include the adrenal hormones: glucocorticoids and adrenaline and noradrenaline.

Actions of the anterior pituitary hormones growth hormone and prolactin

Actions of growth hormone

Growth hormone exerts some direct hormonal effects, but many of its actions are indirect, mediated by another hormone (see Fig. 3.6). The main action of growth hormone is in stimulating the production of a growth factor called insulin-like growth factor 1 (IGF-1, pronounced I-G-F-one) by the liver. The effects of growth hormone are mediated by the growth hormone receptor, which is a member of the recently characterized family of cytokine receptors, as is the IGF receptor (see Chapter 1). Mutations of the gene encoding the growth hormone receptor result in low IGF-1 levels and significantly reduced growth (Laron syndrome).

Effects on growth and metabolism

Both growth hormone and IGF-1 circulate to the tissues to cause growth of nearly every organ and tissue. In pre-pubertal children, before fusion of the epiphyses, growth hormone stimulates long bone growth and is the major hormone responsible for linear growth, although thyroxine is also required for growth to take place (Fig. 3.10). In the absence of growth hormone there is a failure of linear growth (see below).

Growth hormone also has a range of metabolic effects, acting to raise blood glucose and free fatty acid concentrations, while promoting protein synthesis in muscle (Table 3.3). Metabolic effects of growth hormone include:

- *Protein metabolism*: increases amino acid uptake and protein synthesis in muscle.
- *Carbohydrate metabolism*: stimulates gluconeogenesis, decreases peripheral glucose utilization. Generally antagonizes insulin actions.
- *Lipid metabolism*: stimulates release of free fatty acids and glycerol from adipose tissue.

> ### Interesting fact
>
> Some endurance athletes, such as swimmers and cyclists, try to exploit the action of growth hormone on muscle by using it as a performance-enhancing drug. They take injections of recombinant growth hormone in order to increase their muscle bulk and in the hope that it will be less easily detected than anabolic steroids.

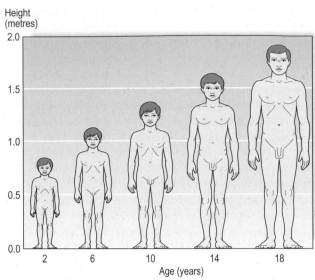

Fig. 3.10
Growth hormone is responsible for the normal increase in height through childhood. In the absence of GH, linear growth is severely limited. A typical height for a 10-year-old boy with a severe GH deficiency would be about 1 metre. However, most cases would be diagnosed at a much earlier age than this.

Table 3.3
Metabolic effects of growth hormone and IGF-1

Metabolic measure	GH	IGF-1
Plasma glucose levels	↑	↓
Hepatic gluconeogenesis	↑	↓
Hepatic glycogenesis	↑	↓
Insulin sensitivity	↓	↑
Glucose uptake (muscle, etc.)	↓	↑
Lipolysis	↑	↓
Protein synthesis (muscle, etc.)	↑	↑

The effects of IGF-1 are very similar to those of insulin as they are each able to bind to both receptors. In general the effects of GH oppose those of insulin. However, both IGF-1 and GH act to increase protein synthesis in muscle.

Actions of prolactin

Receptors for prolactin are located in many tissues including breast, liver, ovary and prostate. Prolactin receptors bind growth hormone with nearly equal affinity. Prolactin is the major hormone of lactation, acting on the oestrogen-primed breast to initiate and maintain lactation. Glucocorticoids have a permissive role in lactation, as does the decrease in oestrogen and progesterone levels postpartum.

Prolactin and growth hormone have a role in the very complex control of breast development in adolescent girls. Oestrogen, progesterone and adrenal steroids are also required, together with insulin and thyroid hormones. Breast development in males is inhibited by testosterone.

In addition, prolactin inhibits ovulation, by inhibiting gonadotropin releasing hormone secretion from the hypothalamus and it is quite normal for a woman who is breastfeeding to have no menstrual cycle until either the child is weaned or the frequency of feeding is insufficient to maintain prolactin levels at high enough concentrations to maintain this inhibitory effect. This effect of prolactin explains why breastfeeding has long been used as natural contraception by many women.

The physiological significance of prolactin receptors in the liver, ovary and prostate is not known. The physiological function of prolactin in men is also unclear.

Disorders of anterior pituitary function: °over-secretion

Pituitary adenomas, tumours of the anterior pituitary that secrete hormones, are relatively uncommon. However, when they do occur they have profound effects on the body. A corticotroph adenoma, secreting ACTH, causes adrenal hyperfunction, resulting in 'Cushing's disease'. A thyrotroph adenoma causes hyperthyroidism, whereas a gonadotroph adenoma affects ovarian and testicular function. These will be considered in more detail in the chapters covering those endocrine systems. In this chapter we will focus on growth hormone and prolactin.

Excess growth hormone secretion

This is most often caused by a secretory tumour (adenoma) of the pituitary somatotroph cells. In children, the effect of excess growth hormone is an increase in linear growth particularly of the long bones, resulting in a condition of extreme height, termed giantism. In adults, excess growth hormone secretion causes acromegaly, a condition easily recognized in its later stages by the characteristic growth of the hands, feet and lower jaw (Fig. 3.11). There is often a coarsening of the facial features, with increased growth of the lips and nose and of the skin above the eyes. The onset of symptoms is usually slow and there is often a delay of several years between the onset of acromegaly and first presentation at an endocrine clinic. The other effects of acromegaly are rather more serious than the visible cosmetic changes. The excess growth hormone also causes growth of the viscera and particularly

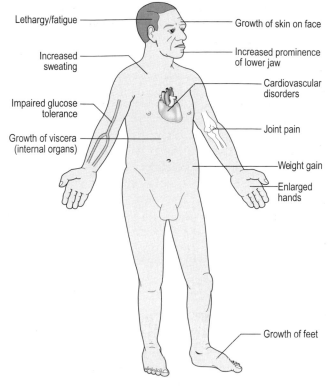

Fig. 3.11
Signs and symptoms of acromegaly (excessive growth hormone secretion in an adult).

affects the heart and cardiovascular system. Metabolic effects include impaired glucose tolerance, which adds to the cardiovascular risk. As a result, premature death from cardiovascular disorders is a significant risk in acromegaly.

high bp

damage blood vessels?

Interesting fact

If you type 'HGH releaser' into an internet search engine, you will find many websites advertising products that are claimed not only to raise your growth hormone levels, but also to stop you from ageing, increase your lean body mass, improve your sex drive and generally bring peace on earth. Using your new-found knowledge of the endocrinology of the pituitary and growth hormone, ask yourself to what extent these claims can be justified. For example, would growth hormone be active if taken orally? Would amino acid mixtures designed to stimulate the pituitary be likely to raise growth hormone above physiological levels? How much money can you make selling these products?

Case note: Explanation of symptoms

The actions of growth hormone and IGF-1 affect all organs and soft tissues (see Fig. 3.11). Long bones are also capable of growth if the growth plates are unfused. This occurs when the tumour develops before puberty, and results in tall stature, or giantism. The effect of excess growth hormone and IGF-1 on the joints is to accelerate arthritis by over-stimulation of cartilage and peri-articular bone. The internal organs also grow and cardiac hypertrophy and high blood pressure result. Sweating is due to growth of the skin and the sweat glands. Growth of the soft tissue surrounding the median nerve results in compression under the carpal tunnel, with bilateral carpal tunnel syndrome causing painful tingling and weakness of the hands, especially at night.

Growth hormone is also one of the three major hormones that counter the action of insulin; the other two are cortisol and glucagon. Thus, impaired glucose tolerance and diabetes are common in acromegaly. This explains Mr Roberts' high glucose concentration.

Growth of the lower jaw and tongue made anaesthesia difficult and the teeth may be loose. Mr Roberts' acromegaly should be controlled or treated before other non-urgent surgery (such as his hernia repair) takes place.

Excess prolactin secretion

Prolactinoma, a prolactin secreting tumour, is the most commonly occurring pituitary tumour. The presence of such a tumour causes hyperprolactinaemia, the condition of excess circulating prolactin concentrations. However, this condition may also result from other causes, particularly as a side effect of drugs that reduce dopaminergic transmission. In women, excess prolactin causes cessation of the menstrual cycle and may cause inappropriate lactation, termed galactorrhoea. In men, prolactin may also cause growth of breast tissue, termed gynaecomastia.

Case history

The class of drugs most likely to cause hyperprolactinaemia is the neuroleptics, dopamine antagonists used to treat psychosis. Mr Green, a 46-year-old man

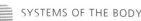

with a long history of psychotic illness, had recently had his neuroleptic medication increased by his GP. At his next outpatient appointment with his psychiatrist, Mr Green appeared to have developed a new symptom. He had always had a variety of false beliefs that various government agencies were plotting against him, but had now become convinced that his GP was trying to turn him into a woman. When asked the standard question 'What evidence do you have for this?', he unbuttoned his shirt to reveal significant gynaecomastia and expressed milk from both breasts. His serum prolactin was 4265 mU/L (normal range <400 mU/L). Three months after changing his neuroleptic medication his serum prolactin was normal, his gynaecomastia had resolved and he was back on speaking terms with his GP.

Disorders of under-secretion of anterior pituitary hormones

Hypopituitarism or under-secretion of pituitary hormones may occur as a result of trauma, infarction or surgical removal of the pituitary gland (hypophysectomy). As the pituitary gland occupies a space confined by bone, the presence of any tumour in the region is likely to cause compression and loss of pituitary function. Although most of the tumours of anterior pituitary cells cause symptoms by over-secretion of a particular hormone, these tumours are also likely to cause a loss of function of other cell types as the tumour compresses the cells. It is also possible to find non-functional tumours that are space occupying and cause an overall loss of anterior pituitary function termed panhypopituitarism.

There is a pattern to the effects of such space-occupying tumours on anterior pituitary function. Growth hormone is usually the first hormone to be lost, with LH/FSH next, and ACTH and TSH being the most resistant to damage. There may be a paradoxical effect on prolactin secretion: if the pituitary stalk is compressed then dopamine inhibition of lactotrophs is lost and prolactin secretion rises.

Panhypopituitarism is a serious condition, resulting in hypotension, hypoglycaemia, lethargy and weakness (Fig. 3.12). The loss of adrenal function due to lack of ACTH can be life threatening (see Chapter 4). There is also a loss of libido and secondary sex characteristics. In children there is growth failure and failure to enter puberty.

Loss of anterior pituitary function means that replacement of some hormones is necessary. In particular, loss of ACTH and TSH results in loss of adrenal

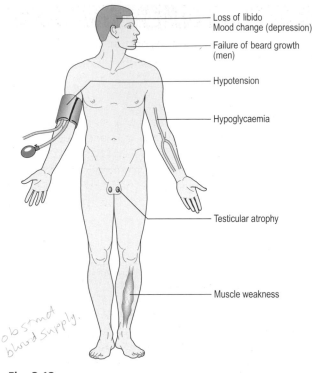

Fig. 3.12
Signs and symptoms of panhypopituitarism.

and thyroid function. As a general rule, it is not the pituitary hormones that are replaced, as these are all large peptides and would require frequent injection. Instead the thyroid hormone, thyroxine, and adrenal steroids are given as these both correct the deficiencies and are active orally.

In the case of the gonadotropins, LH and FSH, secondary sexual characteristics can be induced and maintained by oral administration of sex steroids. However, when a woman with hypopituitarism wishes to conceive, gonadotropins can be used to induce ovulation.

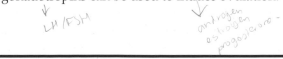

Interesting fact

A very rare, and therefore utterly memorable, cause of hypopituitarism is Sheehan's syndrome. This is caused by a sudden decrease in blood volume or a localized bleed disrupting the hypophyseal portal system. In the bad old days, Sheehan's syndrome was most often associated with blood loss in childbirth. Because the posterior pituitary has a separate arterial supply, Sheehan's syndrome affects only the anterior pituitary, resulting in loss of its hormone secretion.

Tests for hypopituitarism

The first investigation for hypofunction of the pituitary is to measure blood concentrations of the pituitary hormones at 9 am. However, more complex tests are sometimes needed. An insulin tolerance test can be used to check ACTH and growth hormone secretion; a tightly controlled dose of insulin is given to induce hypoglycaemia and the pituitary response is measured by checking levels of ACTH and GH. These hormones are both strongly stimulated by hypoglycaemia. Clearly this is a potentially dangerous test and cannot be used in many patients, such as those with heart disease.

Acromegaly box 5

Case note: Further tests

The anterior pituitary controls other hormonal systems and these may be damaged by pressure or invasion by an anterior pituitary adenoma. An important axis for maintaining blood pressure is the pituitary–adrenal axis. This should be shown to be functioning normally (see Chapter 4) or, if not, be replaced by exogenous glucocorticoids before any surgical treatment of the acromegaly. The serum thyroxine and testosterone levels should also be measured to test the integrity of the pituitary–thyroid and pituitary–gonadal axes respectively.

Occasionally, the prolactin level will be high. This may be because the adenoma secretes both prolactin and growth hormone. However, some tumours block the delivery of dopamine to the normal lactotroph, releasing it from tonic inhibition.

Insufficient growth hormone secretion

The effects of hyposecretion of growth hormone are most significant in children as growth hormone is necessary for normal growth during childhood. However, there are many reasons for failure of growth in children and growth hormone insufficiency is relatively uncommon. In adults, there is increasing evidence that growth hormone is necessary both for the maintenance of a normal body composition and to maintain well-being. In the absence of growth hormone there is an increase in body fat and a loss of muscle strength. Growth hormone deficiency is treated by daily injections of recombinant growth hormone. Growth hormone, like other pituitary peptides used therapeutically, used to be extracted from human or animal pituitary glands, but the possible transmission of prion diseases made this undesirable. At the same time, modern molecular technology has made it possible to produce relatively large amounts of this and other hormones safely.

Acromegaly box 6

Case note: Management

The main treatment of acromegaly is surgical removal of the adenoma. However, although 80% of small tumours (less than 1 cm in diameter) are curable by surgery, only 40% of tumours larger than 1 cm are resectable. This means that additional treatments are needed. Radiotherapy is successful in reducing the size of the adenoma and the levels of growth hormone. However, radiotherapy may take several years for full effect. Medical treatments that may be needed include dopamine agonists and somatostatin analogues. The dopamine agonists work because the somatotroph and lactotroph share a similar cellular lineage and somatotroph adenomas may express dopamine receptors on the cell surface. Somatostatin is a hypothalamic peptide that lowers growth hormone secretion in physiological states. Synthetic analogues of somatostatin (for example, octreotide, which contain eight somatostatin molecules) bind to adenomas and reduce their size and growth hormone secretion in a majority of cases.

The anatomy and relations of the pituitary are vital to the surgical cure of acromegaly. The surgeon approaches the pituitary fossa through the nose and the sphenoidal sinus. The operation must be performed by an experienced surgeon and a particular danger is entry into the cavernous sinuses which are blood-filled venous channels (rather like a sponge) lateral to the fossa. Severe bleeding may result from this error. Radiation therapy may be given, but is planned so that the dose of radiation given to the normal brain structures, in particular the optic chiasm, is as low as possible.

35

Self-assessment case history

A case of lack of periods and breast milk production

Mrs Singh was a 37-year-old woman who had a lack of menstrual periods with breast milk production for the last 18 months. Menarche had been at 13 years of age and her periods had been regular since then. The breast milk was clear and came from both breasts. It was particularly bad at night and would stain her night clothes. She was taking no medication and had been using barrier methods (condoms) of contraception with her husband. She has performed several urine pregnancy tests, which were negative. The examination showed a well woman with bilateral galactorrhoea.

Investigations revealed:

Serum prolactin	4323 mU/L (normal <400 mU/L)
Serum growth hormone	0.5 mU/L (normal <20 mU/L)
Serum free T4	12 pmol/L (normal 9–24 pmol/L)
Serum TSH	1.1 mU/L (normal 0.4–4 mU/L)
Serum cortisol	453 nmol/L (normal 200–600 nmol/L)
Serum LH/FSH	1.1/1.4 mU/L
Serum oestradiol	90 pmol/L (normal follicular phase 200–800 pmol/L)
MRI scan of pituitary	Filling defect of 5 mm in right side of gland

Questions:

① What is the diagnosis?

② What is the mechanism of amenorrhoea?

③ What is the correct management strategy?

Answers see page 147

Extended matching questions

A ACTH (adrenocorticotropin)
B AVP (arginine vasopressin)
C CRH (corticotropin releasing hormone)
D DA (dopamine)
E FSH (follicle stimulating hormone)
F GH (growth hormone)
G IGF-1 (insulin-like growth factor 1)
H LH (luteinizing hormone)
I PRL (prolactin)
J Somatostatin
K TRH (thyrotropin releasing hormone)
L TSH (thyroid stimulating hormone)

For each of the descriptions below, pick the hormone or regulatory factor that best fits from the list above:

① The hypothalamic regulatory factor that is not a peptide.

② The hypothalamic regulatory factor that inhibits growth hormone secretion.

③ The hormone that, along with ACTH, is most resistant to the effects of space-occupying tumours on anterior pituitary function.

④ The hormone that, like FSH, is produced by gonadotroph cells.

⑤ The hormone that is produced as a result of POMC processing.

⑥ The hormone that directly antagonizes the effects of insulin on blood glucose.

⑦ The hormone that mimics the effects of insulin on blood glucose.

⑧ The only pituitary hormone that is under tonic inhibitory control.

Answers see page 150

THE ADRENAL GLANDS

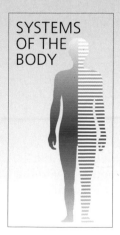

SYSTEMS
OF THE
BODY

Chapter objectives

After reading this chapter you should be able to:

① Describe the structure of the adrenal glands and understand how the inner (medulla) and outer (cortex) parts of each gland have separate functions.

② Describe how the adrenal cortex and medulla are regulated and explain the principles of negative feedback.

③ Describe how the major adrenal hormones are synthesized.

④ Describe the therapeutic uses of glucocorticoids and their unwanted effects.

⑤ Describe the effects of both under- and over-production of adrenal hormones.

⑥ Describe the normal development of the adrenal cortex and explain how abnormal development results in disease.

Introduction

Each adrenal gland is really two quite separate glands. The much larger outer part is the adrenal cortex, which produces steroid hormones (cortisol, aldosterone and androgens), and the smaller inner part is the adrenal medulla, which produces catecholamines (principally adrenaline). Although they function independently, the cortex and medulla share a common blood supply and both have a role in the body's response to stress.

Where to find the adrenal glands

There are two adrenal glands, each situated on the superior pole of the kidneys, embedded in the perirenal fat (Fig. 4.1). They are roughly triangular in shape and each weighs about 4g in the adult. The adrenal cortical tissue totally surrounds the inner medulla, and is arranged in three concentric zones, called the zona glomerulosa, zona fasciculata and zona reticularis (Fig. 4.2).

Interesting fact

Although there are two adrenal glands, if one is damaged or removed the other rapidly increases in size and takes over the function of the damaged gland. So you can lose the function of one adrenal gland without any adverse effects, but losing both adrenal glands may be rapidly fatal unless cortisol is given regularly.

Blood supply

The adrenal glands receive blood from the adrenal arteries, which arise directly from the aorta (see Fig. 4.1). The venous drainage is into a large central vein, which forms the adrenal vein. This drains into the left renal vein from the left adrenal gland, but directly into the vena cava from the right. The importance of the adrenal glands to the body's normal functioning is shown by the fact that, in states of circulatory collapse, the blood supply to the adrenals is preserved. In fact, only the blood supply to the brain is as well protected from interruption.

Interesting fact

The drainage of the short right adrenal vein directly into the inferior vena cava can make it difficult for a surgeon to perform a right adrenalectomy safely. On the other hand, there is a risk of damaging the spleen during a left adrenalectomy. If you're having both adrenals removed, choose your surgeon carefully!

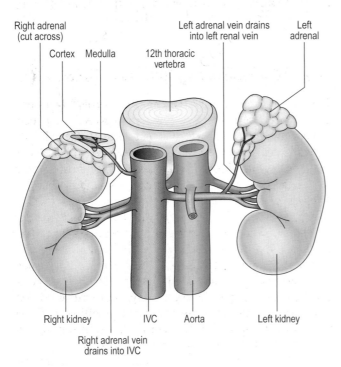

Fig. 4.1
Diagram to show the anatomical relations of the adrenal glands and their blood supply. The arterial supply to the adrenals is via small arterioles that arise directly from the aorta. Note that the right adrenal vein drains directly into the inferior vena cava (IVC), whereas the left adrenal vein drains into the left renal vein.

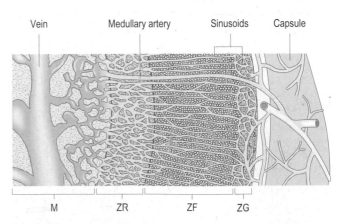

Fig. 4.2
Cross-section through the adrenal gland to show the zonal arrangement of cells, and the blood supply to the gland. ZG = zona glomerulosa, ZF = zona fasciculata, ZR = zona reticularis. Together, these three zones comprise the adrenal cortex. M = adrenal medulla.

Nerve supply

The adrenal medulla is a modified ganglion of the sympathetic nervous system. Instead of noradrenaline being released into the synaptic cleft as a neurotransmitter, it is released into the circulation as a hormone. The adrenal innervation is via the splanchnic nerves, which come from the spinal cord at levels D8–D11.

Embryology of the adrenal gland

As you might expect from their completely different structure and function, the two parts of the adrenal develop from different tissues. The cells of the adrenal cortex are mesodermal in origin, whereas those of the medulla are derived from the neural crest and migrate into the cortical tissue. The fetal adrenal is relatively large, reaching the size of the adult gland at birth. Most of the bulk of the fetal adrenal comprises a special zone, called the fetal zone. The role of the fetal zone appears to be mainly the production of precursor steroids that can be metabolized to oestriol, an oestrogen, by the placenta. This zone disappears rapidly after birth and the adrenal gland decreases in size.

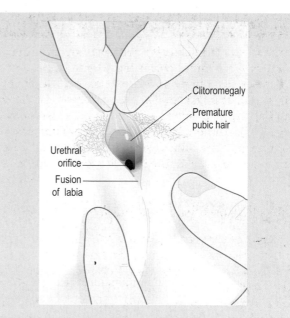

Fig. 4.3
Ambiguous genitalia on a baby girl, characteristic of a severe case of congenital adrenal hyperplasia. Note the fused labia and enlarged clitoris. Note also the pubic hair. (From Chew S L, Leslie D. Clinical Endocrinology and Diabetes: An Illustrated Colour Text. Churchill Livingstone, Edinburgh, 2006.)

Adrenal cortex

Congenital adrenal hyperplasia box 1

Case history

A 4-year-old girl was brought to the paediatric clinic with failure to thrive. The mother reported that her daughter was always thirsty and passed urine frequently. Both height and weight of the child were lower than expected (below the 10th percentile). Pubic hair developed from the age of 3 years and there was an enlarged clitoris with partial fusion of the labial folds (Fig. 4.3). The blood pressure was 70/30 mmHg (normal for a 4-year-old is 90/50 mmHg).
  Blood tests were taken:

Serum sodium 127 mmol/L (normal 135–145 mmol/L)

Serum potassium 5.4 mmol/L (normal 3.5–4.5 mmol/L)

Serum cortisol 128 nmol/L (normal 200–600 nmol/L)

Serum adrenocorticotropic hormone 55 ng/L (normal <50 ng/L)

Lying plasma renin activity 1242 pmol/L/h (normal 230–1000 pmol/L/h)

Serum 17-hydroxyprogesterone 76 nmol/L (normal before puberty <3 nmol/L)

Hormones produced by the adrenal cortex

The adrenal cortex secretes a range of steroid hormones. The most important of these are cortisol (a glucocorticoid) and aldosterone (a mineralocorticoid). Aldosterone is produced exclusively by the cells of the zona glomerulosa, whereas cortisol comes from the zona fasciculata and zona reticularis (see Fig. 4.2). These zones also produce very large quantities of dehydroepiandrosterone (DHEA), a weak androgen that can be converted to both androgens and oestrogens in other tissues of the body. Most of the DHEA is secreted in a sulphated form, as DHEAS. Unlike peptide hormones, the steroids are not stored within the adrenal cells, but instead the gland stores a large amount of cholesterol esters, the substrate for steroid synthesis. These are stored as lipid droplets within the cells, giving the adrenal its classical histological appearance (Fig. 4.4). Normal circulating levels of adrenal hormones are shown in Table 4.1.

Steroid biosynthesis

All adrenal steroids are synthesized from cholesterol by a series of mostly hydroxylation reactions. The

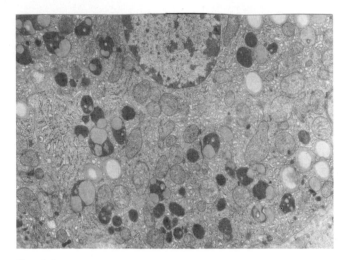

Fig. 4.4
Electron microscopy of the human adrenal zona fasciculata, showing lipid droplets and an abundance of mitochondria in the cells. (From Belloni et al. Journal of Submicroscopic Cytology 1987; 9:657–668, reproduced with permission from Editrice Compositori.)

Table 4.1
Normal circulating concentrations of the major adrenal steroids in the adult

Steroid	Concentration
Cortisol	
8 am	220–660 nmol/L
4 pm	50–410 nmol/L
Dehydroepiandrosterone	0.6–70 nmol/L
Dehydroepiandrosterone sulphate	5.4–9.2 μmol/L
17α-Hydroxyprogesterone	
Women	1–13 nmol/L
Men	1.5–7.5 nmol/L

pathway of adrenal steroid biosynthesis is shown in Fig. 4.5. The enzymes that catalyse steroid hydroxylations are all members of the cytochrome P450 enzyme family. In general, the intermediate products on the pathway are not secreted in significant quantities, and their presence in the circulation can suggest an adrenal disorder (see Congenital adrenal hyperplasia box 1). The major secreted products are highlighted.

Defects of steroid biosynthesis

A deficiency of any of the enzymes involved in steroid biosynthesis will cause a decrease in products downstream of the enzyme and an increase in precursors upstream. Such an enzyme deficiency causes a condition called congenital adrenal hyperplasia, so called because the adrenal gland increases in size as the body tries to increase production of adrenal hormones. The commonest adrenal enzyme deficiency (approximately 90% of cases) affects 21-hydroxylase, which is encoded by the gene *CYP21*. This enzyme converts progesterone to 11-deoxycorticosterone, and converts 17-hydroxyprogesterone to 11-deoxycortisol (see Fig. 4.5). There is, therefore, very low production of both aldosterone and cortisol in patients with 21-hydroxylase (*CYP21*) mutations. The progesterone and 17-hydroxyprogesterone that accumulate are metabolized via the alternative pathway into androgens (Fig. 4.6).

Congenital adrenal hyperplasia box 2

Case note: Establishing the diagnosis

If you look back at the case history box, what do the levels of serum cortisol and serum 17-hydroxyprogesterone suggest? There is a low serum cortisol level, which might indicate primary adrenocortical failure, but there is a raised serum level of 17-hydroxyprogesterone, which is synthesized in the adrenal cortex, so this cannot be a case of failure of the adrenal cortex. This pattern is characteristic of an error in the cortisol production pathway (see Figs 4.5 and 4.6), a condition called congenital adrenal hyperplasia. In 90% of cases this is due to a defect in the gene for the 21-hydroxylase enzyme. This gene defect results in seriously impaired cortisol secretion, but some cortisol is still made. The block in cortisol production results in an accumulation of precursors such as 17-hydroxyprogesterone. The precursors then spill over to make adrenal androgens such as DHEA and androstenedione.

Regulation of steroid production

Cortisol

Cortisol is produced mainly by the cells of the zona fasciculata, with smaller amounts coming from the zona reticularis. Cortisol production is regulated by adrenocorticotropic hormone (ACTH), which, in turn, is regulated by corticotropin releasing hormone (CRH) and arginine vasopressin (AVP) (see Chapter 2). This is the hypothalamo–pituitary–adrenal (HPA) axis (Fig. 4.7). There is a diurnal variation in ACTH production and secretion, and therefore in serum cortisol concentrations, with a peak at 6–9 am (Fig. 4.8). Serum cortisol is therefore usually sampled at 0900 hours. The HPA axis is also stimulated by stress – both by physiological

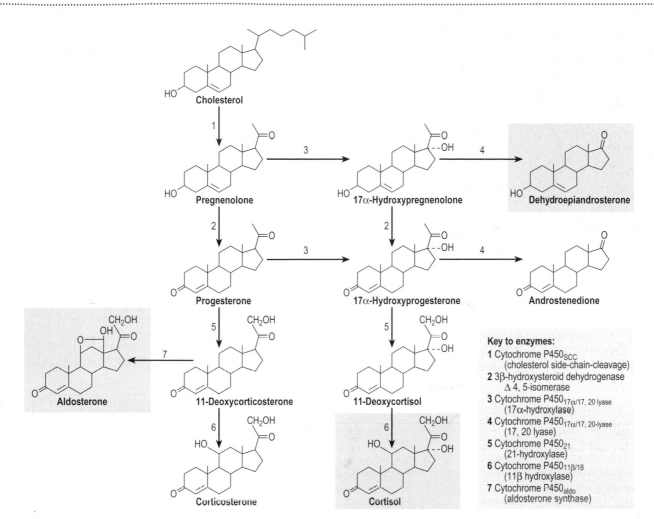

Key to enzymes:
1 Cytochrome P450$_{SCC}$ (cholesterol side-chain-cleavage)
2 3β-hydroxysteroid dehydrogenase Δ 4, 5-isomerase
3 Cytochrome P450$_{17\alpha/17, 20 \text{ lyase}}$ (17α-hydroxylase)
4 Cytochrome P450$_{17\alpha/17, 20\text{-lyase}}$ (17, 20 lyase)
5 Cytochrome P450$_{21}$ (21-hydroxylase)
6 Cytochrome P450$_{11\beta/18}$ (11β hydroxylase)
7 Cytochrome P450$_{aldo}$ (aldosterone synthase)

Fig. 4.5
Pathways of steroid biosynthesis in the adrenal gland. Note that small modifications to the steroid structure produce significant biological differences. Note also that only seven different enzymes produce this range of adrenal steroids. Most of these enzymes are members of the cytochrome P450 enzyme family.

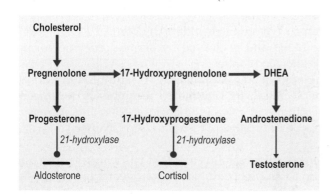

Fig. 4.6
The commonest enzyme deficiency causing congenital adrenal hyperplasia is a defect in 21-hydroxylase, which is a key enzyme in the production of both aldosterone and cortisol. It is not required for androgen biosynthesis, however, so the steroid precursors that accumulate are converted into adrenal androgens.

stressors, such as cold exposure, infection, hypoglycaemia and exercise, and also by psychological stressors, such as exams!

ACTH binds to specific receptors in the plasma membrane and causes an increase in intracellular cyclic adenosine monophosphate (cAMP) production. The ACTH receptor is also known as the melanocortin-2 receptor, and belongs to a family of similar receptors. The major effect of ACTH is to increase the conversion of cholesterol to pregnenolone, which is the rate-limiting step of steroidogenesis. ACTH achieves this effect by increasing the rate of cholesterol delivery to the enzyme, rather than by affecting enzyme activity directly. Because cortisol production is subject to negative feedback regulation (see Chapter 1), decreased cortisol production results in increased ACTH secretion in an attempt to restore cortisol levels. ACTH acts

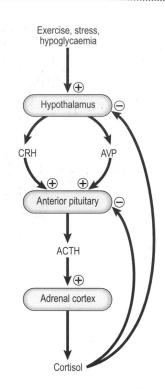

Fig. 4.7
The hypothalamo–pituitary–adrenal (HPA) axis. Activity of this axis is stimulated by stress, hypoglycaemia and exercise. This stimulus causes a release of both corticotropin releasing hormone (CRH) and arginine vasopressin (AVP) from the hypothalamus. These two hormones act together on the corticotroph cells of the pituitary to stimulate adrenocorticotropin (ACTH) release. ACTH acts on the adrenal cortex to stimulate the release of cortisol which, in addition to its other actions, exerts a negative feedback effect on both the hypothalamus and pituitary to decrease activity of the HPA axis.

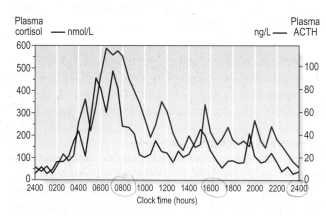

Fig. 4.8
Activity of the HPA axis is subject to diurnal variation, with a peak of activity around 6 am and a nadir around midnight. Note that the increase in ACTH levels precedes the rise in cortisol. Note also that there are secretory peaks during the day, when the axis is stimulated by other inputs (see Fig. 4.7).

both to increase steroid synthesis and to maintain the size and function of the adrenal gland. When cortisol synthesis is impaired, serum ACTH levels can increase significantly, leading to increased adrenal size – adrenal hyperplasia.

Note: It is probably not ACTH itself, but a peptide that is co-secreted with ACTH, that causes the increase in adrenal size.

> **Congenital adrenal hyperplasia box 3**
>
> **Clinical note: Explanation of plasma ACTH result**
>
> Cortisol regulates ACTH secretion by exerting a negative feedback effect on both the hypothalamus and pituitary, so low cortisol levels result in increased ACTH secretion. The effect of ACTH is to drive production of steroid precursors prior to the enzyme defect and induce growth (hyperplasia) of the adrenal cortices.

Aldosterone

Aldosterone is produced exclusively by the cells of the zona glomerulosa. Aldosterone production is regulated principally by the renin–angiotensin system (Fig. 4.9). The renin–angiotensin system is an example of a cascade of protein cleavage steps. Another example (outside the endocrine system) is the clotting cascade. When reduced renal perfusion or a low plasma sodium concentration is detected, the juxtaglomerular cells of the kidney release renin into the circulation. Renin is a proteolytic enzyme that cleaves the large protein secreted by the liver, angiotensinogen, to release angiotensin I, a small peptide. Angiotensin I circulates in the blood and is cleaved by another enzyme, termed angiotensin converting enzyme (ACE) to produce angiotensin II. Angiotensin II stimulates aldosterone secretion by binding to receptors in the plasma membrane of zona glomerulosa cells, and increasing phosphatidylinositol turnover (see Chapter 1).

Note: Angiotensin II is a potent vasoconstrictor in addition to its effects on aldosterone secretion. A first-line treatment for hypertension is an ACE inhibitor, which blocks the formation of angiotensin II. Examples of ACE inhibitors include enalapril, lisinopril and perindopril.

DHEA/S

The adrenal androgens, dehydroepiandrosterone (DHEA) and its sulphated form (DHEAS), are, by

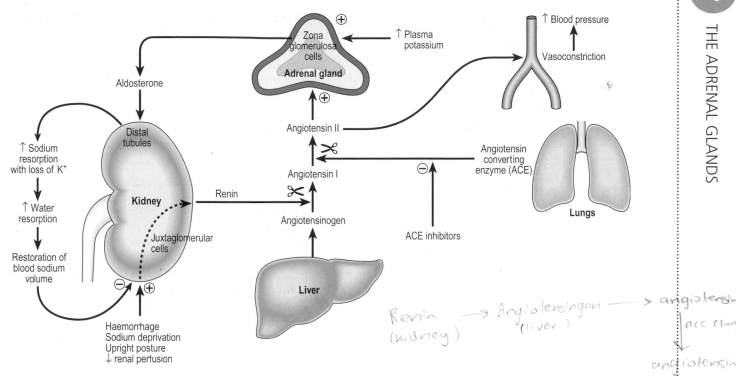

Fig. 4.9

Regulation of aldosterone secretion. Aldosterone has a key role in the maintenance of plasma sodium concentrations and is regulated by the renin–angiotensin system. Briefly, starting at the kidneys, renin is released in response to low renal perfusion (may result from blood loss or postural hypotension) or low plasma sodium ion concentration. Renin is a proteolytic enzyme that cleaves angiotensinogen (a large protein secreted by the liver) to release angiotensin I. The angiotensin I is in turn cleaved by angiotensin converting enzyme (ACE), which is located on the luminal surface of vascular endothelial cells, particularly in the lung. The action of ACE generates angiotensin II, which is both a potent vasoconstrictor and the major stimulus to aldosterone secretion. Aldosterone acts on the distal tubules of the kidney, promoting sodium resorption which leads to restoration of blood volume and sodium concentration.

mass, the major products of the human adrenal cortex. They are not produced in significant quantities in other species. The zona reticularis is the main site of production of adrenal androgens. Although ACTH stimulates adrenal androgen secretion, this is not the whole story as there are many situations in which cortisol and DHEA production are dissociated. This is particularly so in ageing, when DHEA secretion declines significantly while cortisol remains relatively constant through life. In the 1970s and early 1980s there was much research effort directed to finding an 'adrenal androgen stimulating hormone', which has still not been found.

Transport of steroid hormones in blood

Steroid hormones are not naturally very soluble in aqueous solutions such as blood. Many steroid hormones therefore have specific binding proteins, which act to increase their solubility and decrease their metabolism. About 95% of circulating cortisol is bound to plasma proteins, mostly to the specific cortisol binding globulin (CBG), and the rest to albumin. Aldosterone does not have a specific binding protein and is transported in blood with around 60% weakly bound to CBG and plasma albumin.

Actions of adrenal steroids

The major hormonal products of the adrenal cortex are cortisol, aldosterone and adrenal androgens.

Physiological actions of cortisol

The effects of cortisol and similar hormones are termed 'glucocorticoid' because, although cortisol has many actions, its effects on glucose homeostasis were the first to be understood. The term glucocorticoid is now used to refer more properly to hormones that bind to the intracellular glucocorticoid receptor through which cortisol exerts its various effects.

Cortisol has a wide range of effects on glucose homeostasis that oppose, but are generally less important than, the effects of insulin. The overall effects of cortisol on metabolism are to maintain blood glucose levels

Box 4.1

Effects of glucocorticoids

Metabolic effects

- Stimulate mobilization of glucose in liver (glyco-genolysis and gluconeogenesis)

- Stimulate breakdown of fats and proteins

- Increase plasma concentrations of glucose, fatty acids and amino acids

Cardiovascular effects

- Maintain blood volume: increased glucose concentration draws water into blood compartment

- Maintain vascular responsiveness to catecholamines

Other effects

- Anti-inflammatory: inhibit prostaglandin synthesis

- Immunosuppressive

the limbic system, suggesting that cortisol may affect mood, learning and memory.

Cortisol is considered to be a stress hormone because its production is increased in response to a variety of physical and psychological stressors. There is a paradox here though. Cortisol is an essential part of the body's response to stress and in the absence of cortisol even moderate stresses can be fatal. On the other hand, cortisol appears to have a role in both damping down potentially damaging effects and in terminating the stress response.

Physiological actions of aldosterone (Figure 4.9)

The actions of aldosterone are termed 'mineralocorticoid effects' because these actions are on electrolyte balance. Aldosterone acts on the distal convoluted tubule of the kidney nephron and increases sodium reabsorption in exchange for potassium. It brings about this effect by increasing the number of sodium transporter proteins in the nephron. In the kidney, water usually follows the movement of sodium, so aldosterone exerts an anti-diuretic effect.

and liver glycogen stores in the fasting state. Cortisol stimulates protein catabolism in muscle, lipolysis in adipose tissue, and both gluconeogenesis (conversion of non-glucose molecules into new glucose) and glycogenolysis (breakdown of glycogen to release glucose) in the liver (Box 4.1).

Cortisol is able to counteract many of the components of the inflammatory response to tissue injury. It does this by inhibiting the production or action of some of the chemical mediators of inflammation such as histamine, prostaglandins and leukotrienes. Similarly, although cortisol is needed for normal B-lymphocyte function, higher levels of cortisol suppress many aspects of the immune response. Under these conditions cortisol decreases both the number and the effectiveness of T and B lymphocytes. It is likely that the physiological role of cortisol as an anti-inflammatory and immunosuppressant agent is to prevent damage due to excess activity of the inflammatory and immune systems. Both of these effects are utilized therapeutically and are discussed below.

Physiological levels of cortisol are needed for a normal vascular response to noradrenaline. In the absence of cortisol the vasculature is much less responsive to noradrenaline, generally resulting in hypotension. In addition to its negative feedback effects on CRH and ACTH, it is likely that cortisol has important actions on the brain, which are still poorly understood. Glucocorticoid receptors are present throughout the cerebral cortex and are particularly concentrated in

Congenital adrenal hyperplasia box 4

Case note: Salt wasting

In the clinical case, do you think that serum aldosterone levels would be low, normal or high, given the sodium and potassium measurements?

It is likely that plasma aldosterone levels will be low. The high serum potassium and low serum sodium levels are symptoms of mineralocorticoid deficiency. Normally aldosterone acts to raise serum sodium and decrease serum potassium levels, so lack of aldosterone results in low serum sodium and high serum potassium levels. The raised plasma renin activity is a response to the mineralocorticoid deficiency.

The failure to conserve urinary sodium is called 'salt wasting', and is associated with a diuresis, causing polyuria and thirst.

Like other steroid hormones, aldosterone binds to intracellular receptors which are able to interact with DNA to alter the rate of transcription of specific genes (see Chapter 1). The mineralocorticoid receptor has the same affinity for both aldosterone and cortisol, and so binds both hormones equally well. As the concentration of cortisol in blood exceeds that of aldosterone by around 1000-fold it might be predicted that the receptor would always be occupied by cortisol and that aldosterone would be a redundant hormone. The mineralocorticoid receptor does manage to specifically bind aldosterone; it does this by being located together with an enzyme that removes cortisol from the environment of the receptor, thus protecting the receptor from circulating cortisol. The enzyme is 11β-hydroxysteroid dehydrogenase, which converts cortisol to the inactive cortisone, and is found in all mineralocorticoid target tissues.

Interesting fact

A clinical condition, apparent mineralocorticoid excess (AME), may be caused by eating excessive quantities of liquorice. It was discovered that liquorice contains glycerrhitinic acid, an inhibitor of 11β-hydroxysteroid dehydrogenase. The liquorice removes the protection given to the mineralocorticoid receptor, which is then swamped by circulating cortisol. The main symptoms of AME are hypertension with low serum potassium levels.

Congenital adrenal hyperplasia box 5

Case note: Revisiting symptoms and signs

As this child is unable to produce normal physiological concentrations of cortisol and aldosterone she is suffering from symptoms of both glucocorticoid and mineralocorticoid deficiency. She is therefore generally unwell, likely to be hypotensive, and will be unable to tolerate stress. Between feeds her blood glucose level is likely to fall. She is also unable to conserve sodium and has 'salt wasting'. Not all cases of congenital adrenal hyperplasia are associated with salt wasting, as some other adrenal hormones, notably 11-deoxycorticosterone, have mineralocorticoid activity. A deficiency of the 11-hydroxylase enzyme will therefore still cause congenital adrenal hyperplasia, but without the symptom of salt wasting.

Actions of adrenal androgens

The effects of adrenal androgens are generally considered to be significant only in disease states where they are produced in excessive quantities. Under these conditions the adrenal androgens, which are only weakly androgenic compared with testosterone, can have significant virilizing effects. This may result in the development of ambiguous genitalia in female infants with an adrenal disorder, and in hirsutism and acne in women with excess adrenal androgen production. Adrenal androgens may be converted to oestrogens by

the action of aromatase, principally in adipose tissue, providing the only source of oestrogens in post-menopausal women. For this reason there was, briefly in the early 20th century, a trend for removing the adrenal glands in post-menopausal women with a hormone-dependent cancer, such as breast cancer.

Congenital adrenal hyperplasia box 6

Case note: Precocious puberty

In the clinical case, why has the child developed an enlarged clitoris and pubic hair? The presence of pubic hair indicates that this child has developed precocious puberty, which may result from over-production of sex steroids, such as 17-hydroxyprogesterone. The enlarged clitoris is a result of the excess adrenal androgen production, causing abnormal genital development in female babies.

Interesting fact

Although DHEA is conventionally regarded simply as a weak androgen, there is some evidence that it may be more significant than this. Production declines markedly throughout adult life, unlike the other adrenal steroids, and the circulating DHEA concentration is much lower in a variety of disease states. For these reasons DHEA has become a popular anti-ageing remedy, although there is little evidence that taking this steroid has any effects at all on the normal ageing process.

Congenital adrenal hyperplasia box 7

Case note: Treatment and follow-up

The principle of treatment is to give sufficient glucocorticoid to suppress ACTH secretion, so that adrenal androgen production falls within the normal range. The patient will also need fludrocortisone (a synthetic mineralocorticoid).

The patient was treated with hydrocortisone, 5 mg daily in the morning. She underwent surgery to divide the fused labia. When aged 14 years the hydrocortisone was increased to 10 mg daily in the morning to keep pace with her growth. At age 24 years she was referred for genetic counselling as she was now keen to start a family.

What problems do you anticipate and how may these be managed?

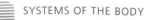
Congenital adrenal hyperplasia is one of the commonest autosomal recessive genetic diseases. Thus, patients with this form of congenital adrenal hyperplasia have mutations or deletions of both copies (alleles) of the 21-hydroxylase gene. In this case the fetus will be a carrier of a mutated allele inherited from the mother. A fetus will have congenital adrenal hyperplasia only if the father is also a carrier of a mutated allele and this is inherited by the fetus. Carriers of mutations in the 21-hydroxylase gene may be found commonly in some populations, and the risk is increased by consanguinity. Before pregnancy is recommended, the partner can be offered a genetic test for common mutations of the gene. If this is not possible or is refused, a biopsy of the placenta (chorionic biopsy) can be performed in the early weeks of pregnancy to test whether the fetus is female. Affected female babies can have severely virilized external genitalia and this can be prevented by steroid treatment (in the form of dexamethasone, which crosses the placenta). Potentially affected babies are tested by measuring the 17-hydroxyprogesterone level in the cord blood at birth, because they are at risk of salt wasting and circulatory collapse.

Therapeutic uses of corticosteroids and disorders of adrenal steroids

Cushing's syndrome box 1

Case history

Mr Jones, a 38-year-old divorced warehouse manager, has suffered from severe asthma since childhood. He has been taking prednisolone, 30 mg orally daily, for the past 18 months. He had become worried after reading about the side effects of steroids and had stopped taking the steroid tablets 3 weeks previously. He was particularly worried about his beer belly, which looked very fat compared with his skinny arms and legs. His sister visited and found him looking very unwell, having been on a long run the day before as the start of his new exercise regime. She immediately called in the general practitioner. On arrival, the GP found Mr Jones to be pale and suffering from nausea and vomiting. Blood pressure was 80/40 mmHg when lying and unrecordable on standing. An ambulance was called and Mr Jones rushed to the nearest accident and emergency department. On arrival, blood was taken and the following plasma concentrations of urea and electrolytes (Us and Es) were obtained:

Serum sodium	127 mmol/L (normal range 136–146 mmol/L)
Serum potassium	4.0 mmol/L (normal range 3.5–5.1 mmol/L)
Serum urea	12.2 mmol/l (normal range 2.5–6.4 mmol/L)

The next morning blood was taken at 0900 hours and the following concentrations were obtained:

Serum cortisol	<50 nmol/L (normal range 200–600 nmol/L)
Serum ACTH	<2 ng/L (normal range 10–50 ng/L)

Mr Jones was treated with intravenous fluids and steroids, and made a rapid recovery. Before discharge the side effects of steroids were discussed and Mr Jones was counselled about the dangers of stopping steroids abruptly.

Disorders of adrenal steroids

Glucocorticoid excess

Cushing's syndrome is the term for any disorder of glucocorticoid excess. It is named after Harvey Cushing (1868–1939), an American neurosurgeon who studied the pituitary gland. There are several possible causes of Cushing's syndrome (Box 4.2). The symptoms of glucocorticoid excess produce a marked change in the appearance of a person, who classically develops a rounded 'moon face' with truncal obesity and muscle wasting in the arms and legs. The skin becomes thinned, with striae developing, and an increased tendency to bruising (Fig. 4.10).

In addition to the alterations in physical appearance, hypercortisolaemia can also result in hypertension, osteoporosis and diabetes mellitus. Wound healing is impaired and there is an increased risk of infection as

Box 4.2

Causes of Cushing's syndrome in order of frequency

① Exogenous corticosteroid administration

② Cushing's disease (hypersecretion of ACTH from the pituitary)

③ Adrenal adenoma

④ Ectopic ACTH production (e.g. from small cell carcinoma)

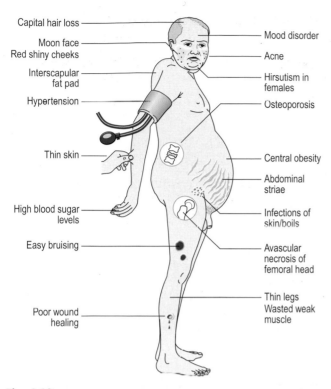

Capital hair loss
Moon face
Red shiny cheeks
Interscapular fat pad
Hypertension
Thin skin
High blood sugar levels
Easy bruising
Poor wound healing

Mood disorder
Acne
Hirsutism in females
Osteoporosis
Central obesity
Abdominal striae
Infections of skin/boils
Avascular necrosis of femoral head
Thin legs Wasted weak muscle

Fig. 4.10
Major features of Cushing's syndrome. Acne, baldness and hirsutism are features of Cushing's syndrome which is due to overactive adrenal glands, as these symptoms result from excess production of adrenal androgens.

the immune system is impaired. There are significant mood disorders associated with Cushing's syndrome. If the disorder is caused by exogenous administration of steroid, this is most commonly associated with elation, whereas excess endogenous steroid is most commonly associated with depression.

Cushing's syndrome box 2

Case note: Diagnosis

What was the cause of Mr Jones' change in body shape? Mr Jones had probably developed Cushing's syndrome as a result of the high dose of prednisolone he was taking to control his asthma. The beer belly and skinny arms and legs he had noticed were truncal obesity and peripheral wasting.

Investigations of glucocorticoid excess
Investigations into glucocorticoid excess are based on an assessment of the feedback of the HPA axis. The

first step is to measure serum levels of cortisol and ACTH. In cases where Cushing's syndrome is caused by exogenous steroids, such as prednisolone, the serum cortisol and ACTH will be undetectable (note that prednisolone is not usually significantly detected by most cortisol assays). In contrast, cortisol levels may be obviously high in patients with an excess of endogenous cortisol. A high serum cortisol with a low ACTH level suggests an adrenocortical tumour secreting cortisol. A high serum cortisol with a detectable serum ACTH level suggests a tumour over-secreting ACTH. ACTH-secreting tumours are usually pituitary adenomas.

The usual principle of endocrinology is to try to suppress a hormone that is thought to be abnormally increased in concentration. In Cushing's syndrome, the commonest test is a dexamethasone suppression test. Dexamethasone is not detected in the blood by the cortisol assay. In a normal patient, intake of dexamethasone at specific doses and times will lead to a suppression of the HPA axis and an undetectable or very low serum cortisol level. If a tumour is over-secreting ACTH or cortisol, the serum cortisol will fail to suppress completely with dexamethasone.

Computed tomography and magnetic resonance imaging are often needed to locate tumours that are over-secreting ACTH or cortisol.

Mineralocorticoid excess (Conn's syndrome)
This is a relatively rare disorder, characterized by hypertension and hypokalaemia. It may be caused by an aldosterone-secreting adrenal adenoma, but idiopathic hyperaldosteronism is also seen. Tumours are usually small and may be removed surgically. The idiopathic disorder is treated with an aldosterone receptor blocker, such as spironolactone.

Adrenal insufficiency
Primary adrenal insufficiency is a failure of the adrenal glands to secrete sufficient amounts of glucocorticoid in response to stimulation. It is also known as Addison's disease, named after Thomas Addison (1793–1860), the English physician who originally classified the disorder. It is usually a disease of slow onset, involving the gradual destruction of adrenal tissue, often by autoimmune disease, or by human immunodeficiency virus (HIV) infection or tuberculosis. The ability of the HPA axis to adapt to loss of tissue is remarkable, and up to 90% of the adrenal cortex can be destroyed before symptoms are seen. However, when the person is exposed to stress, the adrenal cannot respond appropriately and the symptoms of a hypoadrenal crisis develop – *acute adrenal insufficiency* (Box 4.3).

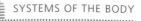

Box 4.3

Signs and symptoms of acute adrenal insufficiency

- Weakness, fatigue, lethargy
- Dehydration, hypotension
- Nausea and vomiting
- Hyponatraemia, hyperkalaemia

Cushing's syndrome box 3

Explanation of clinical presentation

What is the explanation for Mr Jones' clinical presentation? Mr Jones clearly has acute adrenal insufficiency following the abrupt cessation of his steroid therapy. The acute crisis was probably precipitated by the exercise he had taken on the previous day. Although his potassium level was within the normal range, the increased concentration of urea, indicating dehydration, together with the hyponatraemia, point strongly to adrenal insufficiency.

Pharmacological uses of glucocorticoids

The anti-inflammatory and immunosuppressive actions of glucocorticoids are exploited therapeutically to treat a range of disorders. Prednisolone is an example of a synthetic steroid with mainly glucocorticoid actions, so that it acts rather like cortisol. It is often used as an anti-inflammatory agent and is used most widely as a topical preparation for inflammatory skin disorders, or as an inhaled preparation in the prophylaxis of asthma. When used in these forms the risk of side effects is minimized. Glucocorticoids are also used systemically to treat inflammatory diseases, such as systemic lupus erythematosus. There is a significant risk of developing Cushing's syndrome, and of long-term suppression of the HPA axis. All currently available glucocorticoids, except dexamethasone, have some mineralocorticoid activity, and so cause sodium and water retention.

Cushing's syndrome box 4

Case note: Cause of cortisol and ACTH results

One of the major side effects of glucocorticoid therapy is long-term suppression of the HPA axis. When therapy is suddenly discontinued there is a risk of developing the symptoms of adrenal insufficiency.

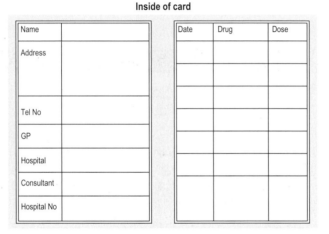

Fig. 4.11
Steroid treatment card. All patients receiving treatment with oral glucocorticoids should be given a steroid treatment card. It is designed to ensure that the patient continues to receive an appropriate level of medication if they are in an accident or undergoing surgery, for example.

Interesting fact

Cortisol is the naturally occurring hormone secreted by the adrenal gland. Cortisol is called hydrocortisone when it is used therapeutically. Both names refer to exactly the same substance.

Steroid treatment card

When patients start a long course of oral glucocorticoid therapy they are given a steroid card (Fig. 4.11) to carry, which details the medication they are taking. Its purpose is mainly to inform doctors who may treat the patient in the event of sudden illness or accident, and so prevent problems of adrenal insufficiency. It also reminds patients of the need to take their medication regularly.

Cushing's syndrome box 5

Case note

How could the GP have helped prevent Mr Jones' illness? If Mr Jones had been given a steroid treatment card he would probably have been more aware of the dangers of stopping his prednisolone without seeking medical advice.

The adrenal medulla

Phaeochromocytoma box 1

Case history

Mrs Smith was a 45-year-old woman who was urgently referred by her GP to the duty medical team at the local hospital, with a 2-week history of sweating and palpitations. She described sudden episodes of rapid heart beating, lasting for 10–15 minutes and occurring at least once an hour. She had been worried that these might be panic attacks as she felt very frightened during these episodes. The GP thought the same until he checked her pulse rate and blood pressure.

On examination Mrs Smith was pale, with a pulse rate of 100/min, and blood pressure fluctuating between 155/105 and 260/165 mmHg. Investigations gave the following results:

Serum sodium	141 mmol/L (normal 136–146 mmol/L)
Serum potassium	3.2 mmol/L (normal 3.5–4.5 mmol/L)
Plasma noradrenaline	12 nmol/L (normal <5 nmol/L)
Plasma adrenaline	6.7 nmol/L (normal <1.5 nmol/L)

The adrenal medulla is the innermost part of the adrenal gland and comprises modified neural tissue. The function of the adrenal medulla is regulated by direct cholinergic input from the splanchnic nerve. The chromaffin cells of the adrenal medulla secrete

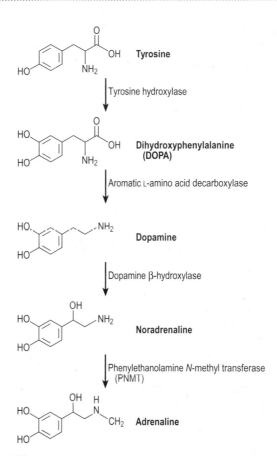

Fig. 4.12
Pathways of catecholamine biosynthesis in the adrenal medulla. The final enzyme in the pathway, PNMT, is regulated by glucocorticoids.

catecholamines, adrenaline (also called epinephrine), noradrenaline (also called norepinephrine) and dopamine, which are synthesized from the amino acid tyrosine (Fig. 4.12). The major product of the adrenal medulla is adrenaline, whereas noradrenaline is more abundant in the central and sympathetic nervous systems. The processes of catecholamine synthesis and release are the same in the adrenal medulla as in the rest of the nervous system. These hormones are part of the classical 'fight or flight' neuroendocrine response. In contrast to most hormones, the effects of catecholamines are very rapid and short lived, with a half-life in plasma of seconds.

Catecholamines activate peripheral adrenoceptors and have a wide range of actions in many different cell and tissue types. Physiologically their major effects are on the cardiovascular system, causing an increase in heart rate and raised blood pressure. They also cause both pupillary and bronchial dilatation, and increased glucose production by the liver. Different receptors mediate these effects. See Table 4.2 for an indication of the effects associated with

4

THE ADRENAL GLANDS

Table 4.2
Effects of adrenoceptor activation

Receptor subtype	Effects	Receptor blockers
α_1	Vasoconstriction Pupillary dilatation	Phenoxybenzamine Doxazosin
α_2	Vasoconstriction	
β_1	Increased heart rate Increased cardiac contractility	Propranolol Atenolol
β_2	Bronchial dilatation Increased hepatic glucose output	

activation of different receptor subtypes, and the drugs that may be used to block these effects. Adrenoceptor blockers are competitive inhibitors of the receptor (i.e. they can be displaced from the receptors by high concentrations of catecholamines).

Excess catecholamine secretion is caused by a neuroendocrine tumour called a phaeochromocytoma. These tumours are usually found in the adrenal medulla, but may occur elsewhere in the sympathetic chain. They are treated by surgical removal, following adrenoceptor blockade with first an α-blocker, followed by a β-blocker.

Phaeochromocytoma box 2

Case note: Establishing the diagnosis

What is the cause of Mrs Smith's signs and symptoms? Mrs Smith had over-secretion of the catecholamines noradrenaline and adrenaline. This is usually the result of a tumour called a phaeochromocytoma.

The overall action of catecholamines is the response to stress ('fight and flight'). The heart beats faster and stronger, and blood pressure and blood sugar levels rise. There is reduced blood flow to non-vital organs, dilatation of the pupils and airways, and increased sweating.

Endocrine hypertension

High blood pressure is classified into essential hypertension or secondary hypertension. The cause of essential hypertension is unknown and most patients fall into this category. However, in approximately 10% of patients hypertension is secondary to an underlying cause. Secondary hypertension is classified into renal, endocrine and vascular causes. Endocrine causes of hypertension include hyperaldosteronism (Conn's syndrome), Cushing's syndrome and phaeochromocytoma.

Phaeochromocytoma box 3

Case note: Treatment

Mrs Smith was treated with an α-adrenoreceptor blocking drug, phenoxybenzamine. A β-adrenoreceptor drug, propranolol, was given a few hours later. The treatment resulted in a steady fall of the blood pressure to 130/80 mmHg.

The likeliest source of high levels of catecholamines in Mrs Smith was a phaeochromocytoma of the adrenal medulla. Therefore, a computed tomographic scan of the abdomen and adrenal glands was carried out, showing a mass in the right adrenal gland. Had the adrenal gland been normal, a tumour might have been found in any of the sympathetic ganglia situated from the base of the skull to the bottom of the pelvis. In Mrs Smith's case, an isotope test was also carried out to confirm that the adrenal mass was a phaeochromocytoma. This scan used a chemical called MIBG ([131]I-*m*-iodobenzylguanidine), which is taken up by catecholamine-producing tissues. This mass took up the radio-isotope MIBG, confirming it to be a phaeochromocytoma.

Several weeks later, and protected by regular treatment with phenoxybenzamine and propranolol, a surgeon removed the right adrenal gland and tumour.

Self-assessment case history

Adrenal incidentaloma

A 45-year-old woman presented with right upper abdominal pain for 3 months. The pain occurred in bouts lasting 2–3 hours. She felt sweaty and nauseated during attacks of pain and would often vomit. She had previously been well and was taking no medication. On examination, she was well but overweight. The face was round and red (plethoric) and the blood pressure was 155/95 mmHg.

A clinical diagnosis of biliary colic due to gallstones was made. An ultrasonographic scan of the liver and gallbladder was requested. This showed stones in the gallbladder. The wall of the gallbladder was thickened. During the scan the radiologist noticed a 4-cm mass in the region of the right adrenal. Computed tomography was performed and confirmed a right adrenal mass. The left adrenal and rest of the abdomen was normal, except for gallstones.

Questions:

① What is the likeliest diagnosis for the adrenal mass?

② What are three alternative, but less likely, diagnoses?

③ What clinical features might suggest the mass was a functioning lesion?

④ What tests would determine whether the mass was functioning or non-functioning?

⑤ If surgical treatment is needed, what is the surgical anatomy of the adrenal blood vessels?

Answers see page 147

Extended matching questions

A   Aldosterone
B   Androstenedione
C   Cholesterol
D   Corticosterone
E   Cortisol
F   Dehydroepiandrosterone (DHEA/S)
G   11-Deoxycorticosterone
H   11-Deoxycortisol
I   17α-Hydroxypregnenolone
J   17α-Hydroxyprogesterone
K   Pregnenolone
L   Progesterone

For each of the descriptions below choose the steroid from the list above that best matches:

① The product of the rate-limiting step of steroidogenesis.

② The major mineralocorticoid secreted by the adrenal cortex.

③ The steroid that shows the most marked age-related decrease in production.

④ The steroid that accumulates in the highest amounts in 21-hydroxylase deficiency.

⑤ The steroid with the greatest effect on increasing blood glucose levels.

⑥ The steroid that is stored in large quantities in adrenal cells.

Answers see page 151

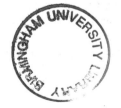

THE THYROID GLAND

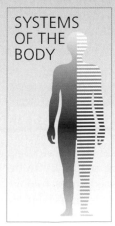

SYSTEMS OF THE BODY

Chapter objectives

After reading this chapter you should be able to:

① Describe the structure of the thyroid glands.

② Describe how thyroid function is regulated and explain the principles of negative feedback.

③ Describe how thyroid hormones are synthesized and explain the significance of peripheral metabolism of thyroxine.

④ Describe the physiological actions of thyroid hormones.

⑤ Describe the effects of both under- and over-production of thyroid hormones.

Introduction

The thyroid gland is located in the neck and is about the shape and size of a bow-tie (Fig. 5.1). The name is derived from the Greek word for 'shield', because the shape of the normal thyroid gland resembles a type of bi-lobed shield. The correct functioning of the thyroid gland depends on a supply of iodine in the diet as the hormones it produces are a modified amino acid containing three or four iodine atoms. The thyroid gland has an important role in regulating metabolism and body weight, and thyroid hormones also play an important role in development.

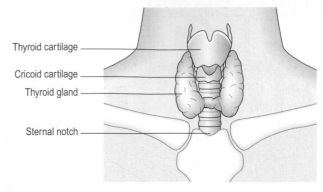

Thyroid cartilage

Cricoid cartilage

Thyroid gland

Sternal notch

Fig. 5.1
Anatomy of the thyroid gland.

Weight loss box 1

Case history

Mr Smith was a 65-year-old man who attended his general practice because of palpitations, sweating and weight loss, despite a good appetite. The symptoms had been present for about 12 months, but began slowly and insidiously. He described the palpitations as rapid and irregular beating of the heart in episodes that lasted from several minutes for up to several hours. The sweating occurred with the slightest exercise and was severe enough to drench his bedclothes at night. His weight had fallen from 75 to 63 kg, despite the fact that his appetite and food intake had increased. His wife complained that he was increasingly irritable and had mood swings.

His medical history was negative and there was no use of medication. On direct questioning Mr Smith admitted to an increased looseness of stools, which were passed twice a day.

On examination, Mr Smith looked well but thin. There was a fine tremor of the hands, which felt hot and sweaty. The pulse was 120 bpm and irregular. There was a mass in the neck (see Fig. 5.2) that rose on swallowing and was firm and nodular. The mass extended behind the notch in the sternum. There was an obvious swelling of both breasts.

Mr Smith's case raises five questions:

① What is the diagnosis?

② Why is knowledge of anatomy essential in his management?

③ What is the aetiology and pathogenesis of the disease?

④ What tests should be requested and how should they be interpreted?

⑤ What are the mechanisms for his symptoms?

Thyroid anatomy

The thyroid gland is located beside the trachea, just below the larynx. It has two lobes, which are flat and oval, one on each side of the trachea, joined by an isthmus across the front of the trachea. The lobes are enclosed with two connective tissue capsules. In between these layers the parathyroid glands are found. There are usually four parathyroid glands, found on the posterior surface of the thyroid gland. The thyroid gland is not usually visible. When the thyroid gland increases in size it forms a characteristic swelling in the neck called a 'goitre'.

Interesting fact

Although there are usually four parathyroid glands, there is a great variation between people. One person was reported to have 104 distinct parathyroid glands, located throughout the neck region. They are usually found attached to the thyroid gland, but may be found in other locations, including within the thyroid itself, or attached to the oesophagus.

What is a goitre?

This term refers to a swelling in the neck, caused by an enlarged thyroid (Fig. 5.2). The normal human thyroid gland is neither visible nor palpable. A thyroid has usually doubled in size in order to be palpable. To be visible, a thyroid has usually increased three-fold in size. Although the presence of a goitre is an indication of likely thyroid disease, it does not tell you anything

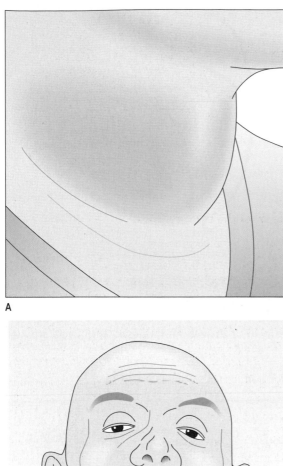

A

B

Fig. 5.2
The appearance of goitre varies tremendously. Goitre can be a relatively small swelling around the neck, looking somewhat like a roll of fat (A) or much larger and more obviously nodular (B).

Iceland, the typical thyroid size is small because the population generally eats a diet rich in iodine. In other regions, normal thyroid size may be four to five times larger. Worldwide, the commonest cause of goitre is iodine deficiency.

So, the presence of a goitre indicates that the thyroid has grown abnormally large and suggests that investigation of thyroid function would be appropriate. The growth may be a result of low thyroid hormone secretion, resulting in high thyroid stimulating hormone (TSH) levels, which then stimulate thyroid growth (see Control of thyroid function), or it may reflect an autonomous growth with excess thyroid hormone secretion. A relatively common cause of an enlarged thyroid is the presence of auto-antibodies that act on the thyroid to stimulate growth and hormone secretion (Graves' disease).

Interesting fact

Some areas, such as Derbyshire, have low naturally occurring levels of iodine in the water supply. Goitre was formerly endemic in these areas and is still sometimes referred to as 'Derbyshire neck'. In the UK, dietary iodine intake is supplemented by the addition of iodide to table salt, making iodine deficiency goitre very rare (see section on Iodine deficiency hypothyroidism).

Blood supply

The thyroid gland has a rich blood supply from the external carotid and subclavian arteries via the superior and inferior thyroid arteries. The rate of blood flow through the gland is controlled by both sympathetic and parasympathetic nerves. The normal rate of blood flow through the thyroid is around twice that of the kidney (at 3 mL per min per g or 30–60 mL per min through the gland), but in disorders involving growth of the thyroid tissue, such as diffuse toxic goitre, may reach 1 L/min in total. This can be detected with a stethoscope: there is an audible bruit over the gland.

Structure of the thyroid

The thyroid gland consists of strands of a single layer of follicular cells surrounding pools of colloid, giving it an unmistakable appearance histologically (Fig. 5.4). On histological examination, when the section is stained with haematoxylin and eosin, the colloid appears pink and relatively homogeneous. The amount of colloid present varies according to the physiological status of the individual: there is

about the underlying cause (Fig. 5.3). The thyroid is usually considered to weigh between 10 and 20 g; however, thyroid size varies hugely between individuals and between different geographical regions. In

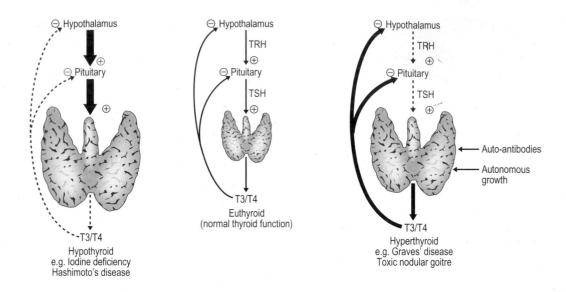

Fig. 5.3

Goitre can result from diseases of both hyperthyroidism and hypothyroidism. In hyperthyroidism the stimulation is either autonomous or from antibodies, leading to thyroid growth and increased hormone output. In these cases TSH levels are extremely low. In hypothyroidism there is very low output of thyroid hormones so TSH levels are high, causing growth of the thyroid gland.

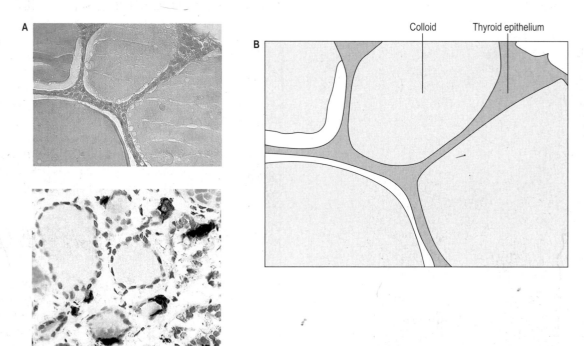

Fig. 5.4

Thyroid histology. (A) Colloid is the smooth material stored in the space between cells. (B) This histological section of a thyroid gland shows thyroid follicles, with C cells showing as darkly staining cells in the parafollicular space. These are the calcitonin secreting cells. (From Chew S L, Leslie D 2006 Clinical endocrinology and diabetes: an illustrated colour text. Churchill Livingstone, Edinburgh.)

more colloid present when the gland is inactive and almost none when the individual is iodine deficient. Amongst the follicular cells are scattered C cells, which secrete calcitonin. These are larger than the follicular cells.

Synthesis of thyroid hormones

The thyroid gland makes active thyroid hormones by adding iodine residues to the amino acid tyrosine. Iodine is taken up into the follicular cells of the thyroid

Case note: Why knowledge of anatomy is essential in his management

The fact that a neck mass is of thyroid origin can be shown by clinical examination and a knowledge of the anatomy and relations of the thyroid. The thyroid gland is wrapped in a layer of tissue called the pre-tracheal fascia, which is inserted into the trachea (see Fig. 5.1). Thus, thyroid masses grow around the trachea and move with the trachea when the patient is asked to swallow. The trachea may become narrowed and even occluded by a thyroid mass, a potential medical and surgical emergency. The surgical anatomy of the thyroid gland is important in operations to remove the thyroid and in counselling patients about the risks of such procedures. The surgeon may have to contend with retrosternal extension, recurrent laryngeal nerve and parathyroid injury. The trachea often descends behind the sternum in older patients owing to a kyphosis of the neck; this is easily appreciated if the cricoid cartilage is found to be at the sternal notch.

Mr Smith's chest radiograph (Fig. 5.5) confirms that the thyroid is exerting pressure on the trachea and indicates a role for surgical removal once the overactive thyroid state has been fully controlled by medication.

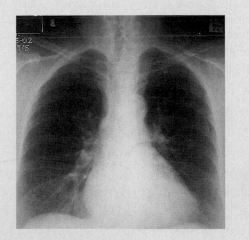

Fig. 5.5
Chest radiograph of Mr Smith showing tracheal deviation. The increased size of his thyroid has exerted pressure on the trachea, causing it to be shifted to one side. (From Chew S L, Leslie D 2006 Clinical endocrinology and diabetes: an illustrated colour text. Churchill Livingstone, Edinburgh.)

by a sodium/iodide symporter, which uses the sodium ion concentration gradient to enable the cells to take up iodide against a concentration gradient. The follicular cells also synthesize a large protein, rich in tyrosine residues, called thyroglobulin. Both the iodide and thyroglobulin are secreted into a pool of colloid, which is surrounded by follicular cells. On the luminal (next to the colloid) surface of these cells there is an enzyme, called thyroperoxidase, which catalyses the reaction between pairs of tyrosine residues and the iodide, and adds four iodides to each pair of tyrosines (Figs 5.6 and 5.7). This iodinated colloid acts as a reserve of thyroid hormone for the body. Normally the thyroid contains 5–6 weeks' supply of hormone. When the follicular cells are stimulated to produce thyroid hormones, droplets of the colloid are taken up by endocytosis into the cell, to form vesicles. These vesicles fuse with lysosomes, which contain enzymes that cut the thyroglobulin to release thyroxine.

Thyroxine and T3: the thyroid hormones

The thyroid gland releases two hormones into the blood, thyroxine (tetra-iodothyronine, also called T4) and T3 (tri-iodothyronine). Their structures are shown in Figure 5.7. The active hormone is T3, but thyroxine can be converted to T3 in many tissues of the body, by a process called 'peripheral deiodination'. The thyroid gland and the mechanism of peripheral de-iodination can also produce an inactive form of T3, called 'reverse T3' (see Fig. 5.7). Thyroid hormones are fat soluble and must therefore circulate in blood attached to a protein, thyroid binding globulin (TBG).

Control of thyroid function

The thyroid gland is regulated by a peptide hormone secreted from the anterior pituitary, quite sensibly called thyroid stimulating hormone (TSH). The control of thyroid hormone secretion is shown in Figure 5.8. This is a classical hypothalamic–pituitary axis, with thyroid hormones exerting negative feedback control of the axis. There is also inhibitory input from other hormones, including somatostatin and glucocorticoids. Examples of stimuli that increase activity of the hypothalamo–pituitary–thyroid axis include cold exposure, exercise and pregnancy.

Functions of thyroid hormones

In the tissues, thyroid hormone diffuses across the plasma membrane into the cell and binds intracellular

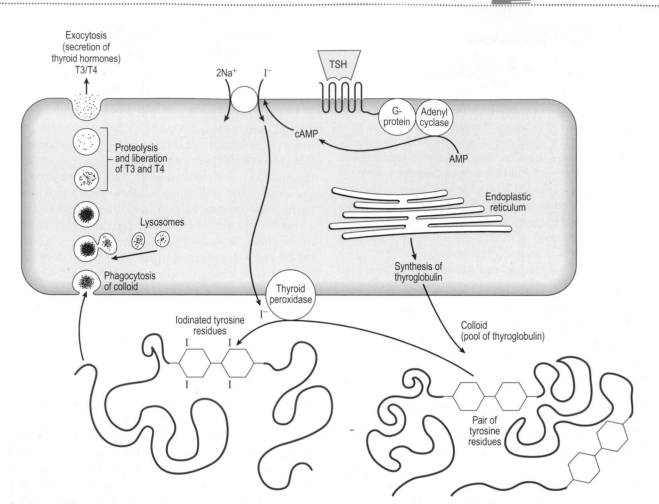

Fig. 5.6

Synthesis of thyroid hormones. Iodine is actively concentrated by thyroid cells. An enzyme called thyroperoxidase catalyses the addition of iodine to the tyrosine residues in thyroglobulin, a large protein, rich in tyrosine residues, that is synthesized in thyroid cells. The iodinated thyroglobulin is stored in the thyroid in the form of 'colloid'. In response to TSH stimulation, portions of the colloid are taken back into the thyroid cell by phagocytosis and pairs of iodinated tyrosine residues (thyroxine) are released into the circulation. Anti-thyroid drugs, such as carbimazole, act by inhibiting thyroperoxidase activity. AC, adenylyl cyclase; cAMP, cyclic adenosine monophosphate.

Weight loss box 3

Case note: Investigations

Mr Smith's doctor requested a thyroid function test, estimation of sex hormone binding globulin (SHBG) level, thyroid auto-antibodies, and an ECG.

The following test results were obtained:

Free T4	28 pmol/L (normal 9–25 pmol/L)
TSH	<0.01 mU/L (normal 0.4–4 mU/L)
Total T3	10.8 nmol/L (normal 1.2–2.2 nmol/L)
SHBG	135 nmol/L (normal male 25–55 nmol/L)
Thyroid microsome autoantibodies	Negative
ECG	Atrial fibrillation, rate 140 bpm

Interpretation of thyroid function test results

Mr Smith has abnormally high serum thyroxine (T4) and tri-iodothyronine (T3) levels. The normal thyroid produces mostly (80%) T4, and this is converted by loss of one iodine molecule (called de-iodination) to the active T3 by the tissues. The production of T4 is normally under the control of the pituitary hormone TSH. However, in Mr Smith's case, the thyroid nodules are autonomously making large amounts of T3 and some T4. The TSH is therefore inhibited by negative feedback effects of the thyroid hormones.

The thyroid hormones are stimulating the liver to produce SHBG, which is a marker of thyroid state and

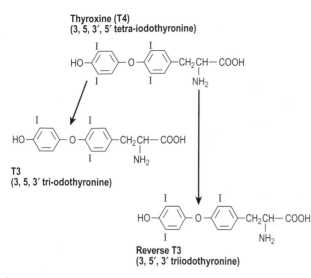

Thyroxine (T4)
(3, 5, 3′, 5′ tetra-iodothyronine)

T3
(3, 5, 3′ tri-odothyronine)

Reverse T3
(3, 5′, 3′ triiodothyronine)

Fig. 5.7
Structure of thyroxine and T3. These small lipophilic hormones act by binding to intracellular receptors. Thyroxine (T4) is converted to T3 or reverse T3 by de-iodination in peripheral tissues. Reverse T3 is inactive.

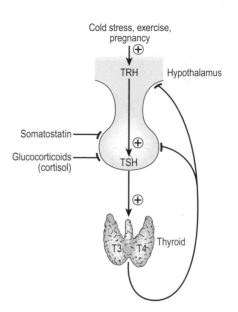

Fig. 5.8
The hypothalamo–pituitary–thyroid axis.

which binds and inactivates testosterone. The reduction in testosterone action allows an increased effect of oestrogen on breast tissue, causing hyperplasia. The latter fact explains the swollen breast tissue (called gynaecomastia).

An alternative diagnosis may have been autoimmune thyroid disease, in which thyroid autoantibodies are usually present. Thus, the negative thyroid autoantibodies result supports a diagnosis of toxic nodular goitre as opposed to Graves' disease.

The ECG confirms atrial fibrillation, which is a dangerous cardiac complication of thyrotoxicosis. Atrial fibrillation is a classical complication and carries a risk of stroke. Clots can form in the fibrillating atria and may move into the arterial system (a process called embolization).

Weight loss box 4

Case note: Establishing the diagnosis

Mr Smith is suffering from the effects of an excess of thyroid hormone (thyrotoxicosis), caused by a toxic nodular goitre. A goitre is an enlarged thyroid gland (see above). Most people over 40 years have small thyroid nodules detectable by high-resolution ultrasonography. Some of these nodules, in a minority of patients, will grow sufficiently to be seen or felt. Thyroid nodules may grow beyond normal control mechanisms and become autonomous. Autonomy means that the nodules produce thyroid hormones independently of control by the pituitary gland. Thus, the TSH level may fall while the nodule continues to produce thyroid hormones. Autonomous thyroid hormone production from the nodule then insidiously worsens until finally an excess of circulating thyroid hormones produces symptoms of thyrotoxicosis. Such thyroid glands are called 'toxic' for this reason.

receptors. Once bound to their ligand, the receptors stimulate transcription of several genes.

Thyroid hormones act on receptors found in the nucleus of target cells. So these hormones act in the same way as steroid hormones, by directly affecting the rate of transcription of certain genes. Both thyroxine and T3 are able to bind to thyroid hormone receptors, although most of the effects of thyroid hormones are mediated by T3.

Thyroid hormones have a range of subtle effects in the body. Although the direct effects of these hormones on particular tissues or cells may be subtle, both thyroid hormone insufficiency and excess result in significant disease.

Like glucocorticoids, thyroid hormones do not have a single specific target tissue, but their receptors are found in most cells and tissues of the body. Although it is possible to state that cells need thyroid hormones to maintain their appropriate function, it has been difficult to identify their physiological effects. One of the main actions of thyroid hormones, however, is to

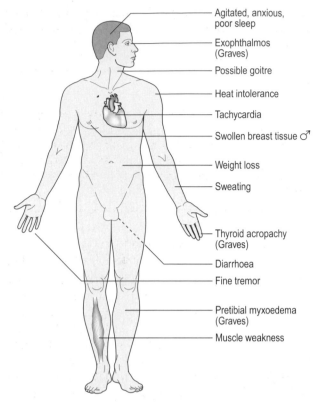

Fig. 5.9
Signs and symptoms of hyperthyroidism (thyrotoxicosis).

produce an increase in basal metabolic rate and an increase in the oxygen consumption of cells. Thyroid hormones also act to alter responsiveness of cells to other hormones, especially to catecholamines.

During fetal development and early childhood, thyroid hormones have an important role in neural development. Up to 11 weeks of fetal life, the developing fetus depends on the small amount of thyroxine that passes across the placenta from the maternal circulation. Although there is a significant increase in circulating maternal thyroid hormones (see Chapter 7, section on pregnancy), this is accompanied by an increase in plasma binding globulin, so the concentration of free thyroxine is unchanged.

Effects of excess thyroid hormone secretion – thyrotoxicosis (Fig. 5.9)

Thyroid hormones have effects on most tissues of the body, so the effects of excess thyroxine are global. The increased basal metabolic rate makes the person feel hot and sweaty. This is often noticed by the individual as heat intolerance, feeling hot even in cool temperatures. As glycolysis increases, there is increased demand for glucose, so both weight loss and increased appetite are often seen together. The general catabolic state leads to a loss of muscle mass, which leads to

muscle weakness. This is most noticeable in the large muscles around the hip and shoulder.

Thyroid hormones alter the actions of other hormones, especially the catecholamines, so tachycardia (increased heart rate) is seen. The tachycardia may be associated with atrial fibrillation, heart failure and death. Thyrotoxicosis is therefore a significant illness and should be treated promptly. The enhanced adrenergic effect also causes a peripheral tremor – typically a fine tremor of the hands. There are effects on mood, and excess thyroid hormones can cause elation, restlessness, anxiety or irritability. Excess thyroid hormones can also cause diarrhoea, by directly stimulating gut motility, and menstrual irregularities. The menstrual irregularities arise from a combination of weight loss and direct effects of the thyroid hormones on hypothalamic and pituitary hormones.

Weight loss box 5

Case note: Explanation of symptoms

Mr Smith's symptoms are due to an excess of thyroid hormones (thyrotoxicosis):

- Increased metabolic rate causes sweating, heat intolerance and weight loss despite good appetite.
- Effects on skeletal muscle may cause proximal myopathy.
- Effects on cardiac smooth muscle may cause atrial fibrillation (causing palpitations).
- Effects on brain cause agitation and labile mood.
- Effects on β-adrenoceptors cause increased heart rate and peripheral tremor.

Disorders of the thyroid: hyperthyroidism

The diagnosis of an 'overactive thyroid' is relatively common. It has been estimated that up to 5% of British women have hyperthyroidism at some time in their lives, with half of these women having thyroid stimulating antibodies in their blood. Thyroid disorders are much less common in men. Hyperthyroidism results in a clinical condition called thyrotoxicosis, in which the levels of circulating thyroid hormones are so high that they cause symptoms.

The two commonest causes of thyrotoxicosis are toxic nodular goitre and Graves' disease. In both of these diseases thyroid function is increased in the absence of stimulation from the pituitary. In toxic nodular disease there is an autonomous nodule in the thyroid gland that slowly increases thyroid hormone production.

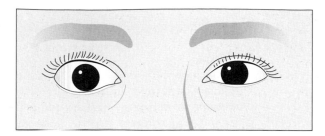

Fig. 5.10
Graves' exophthalmia (proptosis). In this case only one eye is affected. A combination of fat deposition behind the eyes and retraction of the eyelids causes this effect, which is characteristic of Graves' disease and is probably an effect of the antibodies rather than the increased levels of thyroid hormones.

Graves' disease is an autoimmune condition in which auto-antibodies are made against the thyroid and stimulate the TSH receptor. The auto-antibodies take over control of the thyroid from TSH. Graves' disease is part of a spectrum of organ-specific autoimmune disease, including conditions such as pernicious anaemia. Both toxic nodular goitre and Graves' disease cause the symptoms of excess thyroid hormone secretion (see above), but additional signs and symptoms are seen in Graves' disease. In particular, effects on the eye are seen, upper lid retraction and exophthalmos being most noticeable (Fig. 5.10). Graves' disease is also associated with vitiligo (patchy skin depigmentation), myxoedema (thickening of the skin on the lower legs) and finger clubbing.

Interesting fact

Thyroxine is available over the internet as an 'aid to weight loss'. A quick glance at the effects of excess thyroid hormones should be enough to convince you of the foolishness of this course of action. Thyroxine supplements should be taken only on the advice of a qualified doctor.

Treatment of thyrotoxicosis

Thyroid hormones are derived from the amino acid tyrosine, by adding iodine molecules. This process can be blocked by anti-thyroid drugs, for example carbimazole. Thyroid hormones influence all tissues, and the tissue effects may take weeks to resolve after the introduction of drugs such as carbimazole. Another treatment of thyrotoxicosis is to use radioactively labelled iodine. The thyroid gland is the only organ in the body to trap iodine with great efficiency and thus radioiodine will localize nearly exclusively to the thyroid and will painlessly and safely destroy the thyroid tissue over a period of several weeks to months.

Weight loss box 6

Case note: Treatment

There are several aims in treating Mr Smith:

① Control of thyroid hormone levels

② Treatment of atrial fibrillation and its complications

③ Long-term treatment of the nodular goitre.

Mr Smith was started on the anti-thyroid drug, carbimazole. However, it usually takes several weeks for the drug to be fully effective and the tissue effects of thyrotoxicosis may take weeks to resolve after the introduction of anti-thyroid drugs. Thus, the β-adrenoceptor blocking drug, propranolol, was also started. High thyroid hormone levels act together with catecholamines to stimulate the heart and tissues. Blocking the β-adrenoceptor may improve some symptoms in many patients.

The treatment of Mr Smith's atrial fibrillation is essential as there is a risk of clot formation in the heart with embolization to the brain and other parts of the vascular tree. Mr Smith was therefore given warfarin (an anticoagulant) to reduce the risk of clots.

Nodular goitres may be treated by surgery or radioactive iodine. A treatment plan for Mr Smith was made which included the use of radioactive iodine several weeks after he had been rendered clinically and biochemically euthyroid by drug treatment.

Effects of thyroid hormone insufficiency – myxoedema (Fig. 5.11)

The symptoms of hypothyroidism in adults develop only slowly, over a long period of time. Symptoms are often of general tiredness and lethargy. There may be weight gain despite poor appetite. Hypothyroidism often causes depression in about 50% of cases, as well as cognitive impairment, a general sluggishness of

Case history

Ms Cooper, a 54-year-old bank executive, was referred to psychiatry outpatients for assessment of her depression, which was resistant to treatment. She had felt increasingly depressed over the past 6 months and had presented to her GP 6 weeks earlier, whereupon treatment with an antidepressant had been started. This had had no effect on her mood and other symptoms, to the point where Ms Cooper was becoming suicidal. She described low mood, lack of energy and lack of enjoyment – the three core features of depression.

Ms Cooper had been unable to work for the past month and had considerable difficulty concentrating. She was very pessimistic about the future and felt guilty that she was unable to 'snap out of it'. Her appetite was decreased, but she had not lost weight, despite eating much less than usual. She reported increased sleep at night and daytime sleepiness.

Ms Cooper had no history of psychiatric disorder or other significant illness. There was no family history of depression or other psychiatric disorder, but Ms Cooper's mother had a history of hypothyroidism.

On direct questioning, Ms Cooper described how she had been feeling tired and run down for over a year and that she had become intolerant of cold, wearing thick winter clothing on a warm August day. Normally she was very energetic, with a busy lifestyle, and was particularly distressed that she had had to gradually give up more and more of her activities due to her tiredness and lack of concentration.

A thyroid function test was requested. The results were:

Free T4   6.7 pmol/L (normal 9–25 pmol/L)

TSH   112 mU/L (normal 0.4–4 mU/L)

Ms Cooper was started on 50 μg thyroxine per day and was stabilized on 125 μg per day.

Within 3 weeks of starting thyroxine treatment her mood had lifted, tiredness decreased, she felt less sleepy and her appetite had increased. Some 3 weeks later she had made a full recovery, returned to work and started some other activities. At this point the antidepressant medication was stopped.

This case raises the question: Why was a thyroid function test requested rather than alternative forms of antidepressant treatment?

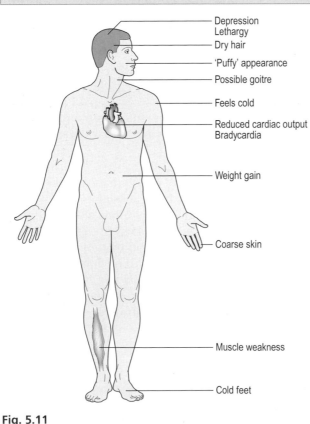

Depression
Lethargy
Dry hair
'Puffy' appearance
Possible goitre
Feels cold
Reduced cardiac output
Bradycardia
Weight gain
Coarse skin
Muscle weakness
Cold feet

Fig. 5.11
Signs and symptoms of hypothyroidism.

intellectual process. There is reduced cardiac output and the pulse rate is slow.

Causes of thyroid hyposecretion

Globally, hypothyroidism is most commonly caused by dietary iodine deficiency, although this is not usually seen in Western societies. There are also auto-immune causes, such as Hashimoto's thyroiditis, caused by auto-antibodies directed against thyroglobulin or thyroid peroxidase. These antibodies cause progressive destruction of the thyroid gland. Hypothyroidism may also result from insufficient pituitary secretion of TSH, although this is uncommon.

Iodine deficiency hypothyroidism

The thyroid gland has an absolute requirement for a supply of iodine in the diet. The World Health Organization recently reported that 30% of the world's population is at risk of iodine deficiency disorders. Children born to severely iodine-deficient mothers have a condition of severe mental retardation termed cretinism, which is the result of a lack of thyroid hormones. At the start of the 21st century, 750 million people were reported to suffer from iodine deficiency goitre. Some 43 million people have brain damage resulting from a deficiency of iodine and therefore of thyroid hormones. This is the commonest preventable cause of brain damage in the world today.

Congenital hypothyroidism

In children hypothyroidism is very serious and can result in severe brain damage. Congenital hypothyroidism occurs in about 1 in 4000 children born in the UK. This relatively high incidence, combined with the seriousness of the condition and its simple treatment once detected, mean that a national screening programme has been introduced in the UK. All babies born in the UK have a heel-prick blood test when they are about 7 days old. The blood spot is tested for thyroid hormones and thyroxine treatment is started if there is evidence of hypothyroidism. There is good evidence that thyroid hormone replacement prevents the consequences of hypothyroidism in these children, although it does not correct any damage that occurred before birth.

Treatment of hypothyroidism

Thyroxine replacement is given to treat hypothyroidism. It is active orally and so can be taken in tablet form. The long half-life of thyroxine in blood means that it can be taken once daily. The aim of treatment is to bring the patient into a 'euthyroid' state. This is best judged, in patients with an intact pituitary, by measuring plasma TSH levels. The aim of treatment is to keep the plasma thyroxine at a level where TSH is just suppressed below about 4mU/L. This usually requires 'titration' of the dose of thyroxine (i.e. a process of trial and error).

Interesting fact

One of the simplest and most effective measures put in place to improve public health across the world has been the addition of iodine to table salt to prevent the mental retardation caused by thyroxine deficiency. Iodine and foods rich in iodine have long been known as a treatment for goitre – in Chinese medicine seaweed is used. Since the early 20th century salt manufacturers have added iodine, usually in the form of potassium iodide, to table salt. Although the World Health Organization strongly supports iodization of salt, it is not a universally popular measure.

Self-assessment case study

A patient with a large goitre

Mrs Zabedic was a 75-year-old woman who was brought to the emergency department because of breathlessness and making a musical sound whenever she breathed. The symptoms had started suddenly 3 days earlier and had since worsened. During this time she was unable to swallow solid food. She had travelled to the UK 5 years earlier to live with her son and had spent all her life in Africa. She had no past medical history and was taking no medications, and had never smoked or taken alcohol. On direct questioning she had noticed a swelling in the neck for years, but never had symptoms from it until 3 days earlier.

The examination showed a breathless elderly but fit woman. There was a lumpy (nodular) mass in the neck from the cricoid cartilage that descended behind the sternal bone. The mass rose with swallowing. The veins of the neck were distended. When she took a breath in a musical sound was generated (a clinical sign called stridor).

The patient was prescribed oxygen. Blood tests, chest radiography and computed tomography were performed. Among the blood tests results were: free T4 level of 22 pmol/L (normal 9–25 pmol/L) and TSH 1.2 mU/L (normal 0.4–4 mU/L). A surgeon was called to see Mrs Zabedic and he recommended an urgent neck exploration and removal of the mass. After consent of the patient, the operation went ahead. On the second day after the operation, the patient was no longer breathless. However, she had developed tingling and stiffness in both hands.

Questions:

① List the anatomical structures that were compressed by the neck mass resulting in the symptoms experienced by Mrs Zabedic.

② What is the likeliest diagnosis of the neck mass?

③ Which of the following terms best describes the thyroid function of Mrs Zabedic: euthyroid, hyperthyroid or hypothyroid?

④ List the structures that may be damaged by surgical removal of the neck mass.

⑤ What hormonal deficiency may explain the symptoms on the second day after surgery?

Answers see page 147

Extended matching questions

A   Cricoid cartilage
B   Eyes
C   Fingers
D   Heart
E   Inferior thyroid artery
F   Oesophagus
G   Kidneys
H   Parathyroid glands
I   Recurrent laryngeal nerve
J   Skin
K   Superior thyroid artery
L   Trachea

For each of the descriptions below, choose the appropriate structure from the list above:

① What non-endocrine structure is most likely to be damaged during thyroid surgery?

② What is likely to have been damaged during thyroid surgery when a patient complains of tingling in both hands after the operation?

③ What structure may allow the extent of thyroid enlargement to be visualized on chest radiography?

④ The effects of thyrotoxicosis on what structure may often be alleviated by propranolol?

⑤ What structure is affected by the exophthalmos associated with Graves' disease?

⑥ What structure is affected by the myxoedema associated with Graves' disease?

Answers see page 151

HORMONAL CONTROL OF REPRODUCTION PART I: MALE REPRODUCTIVE SYSTEM

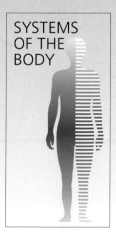

SYSTEMS OF THE BODY

Chapter objectives

After reading this chapter you should be able to:

① Describe the structure and function of the testes.

② Explain the control of steroid hormone production by the testes.

③ Describe the hormonal regulation of spermatogenesis.

④ Understand the endocrine abnormalities that may affect men's sexual health.

The testes (Fig. 6.1) are the male gonads (the singular is testis). The testes have two key functions. The first is the production of gametes, called sperm, by a process called spermatogenesis. The second function is the synthesis of male sex hormones, which are a class of steroid hormones called androgens. The principal male sex steroid is testosterone.

Where are the testes?

The testes are located outside the abdominal wall, in a sac called the scrotum (see Fig. 6.1). During fetal life the testes develop within the abdomen, and descend to the scrotum during the later stages of fetal development. The location of the testes is significant; spermatogenesis requires a temperature somewhat lower than normal body temperature and this is achieved by locating the testes in the scrotum. In an adult male each testis is usually 20–25 mL in volume. In a small proportion of boys (approximately 3% of baby boys delivered at term, but 30% of pre-term boys) one testis has failed to descend fully into the scrotum, a condition known as cryptorchidism (meaning 'hidden testis'), which is treated surgically. The route of descent of the testes from the abdomen into the scrotum is shown in Figure 6.2.

Interesting fact

The fact that a relatively low temperature is required for spermatogenesis has led to the myth that taking a hot bath before sexual intercourse diminishes a man's fertility enough to act as a contraceptive. Given that the process of sperm maturation takes 70 days, it would need to be a *very* long hot bath!

Like many myths, this one has its basis in fact. Over the longer term, conservative measures like wearing looser clothing and avoiding hot baths can improve fertility in sub-fertile men.

What are the testes?

The testes are made up of two functional parts: the seminiferous tubules and Leydig cells (Fig. 6.3). The bulk of the testicular volume (approximately 90%) is made up of seminiferous tubules, which give the testis its lobular appearance. Each seminiferous tubule would be about 60 cm long if stretched out, but luckily is tightly coiled within the testis. The seminiferous tubules are the location of spermatogenesis. The second

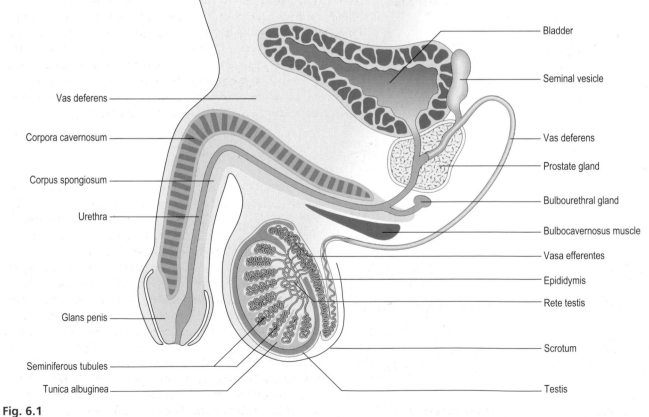

Fig. 6.1
Structure of the male reproductive system.

A

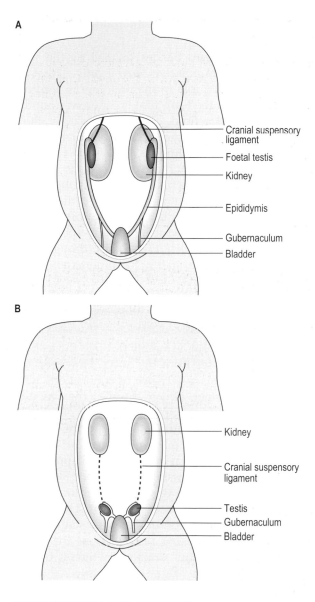

Cranial suspensory ligament
Foetal testis
Kidney
Epididymis
Gubernaculum
Bladder

C

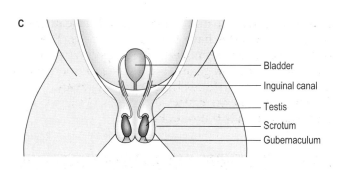

Bladder
Inguinal canal
Testis
Scrotum
Gubernaculum

B

Kidney
Cranial suspensory ligament
Testis
Gubernaculum
Bladder

Fig. 6.2
Descent of the testes from their original site adjacent to the kidney into the scrotum. This is a complex process and the testis can become 'stuck' at almost any point during its descent (A). The fetal testis is held next to the kidney by the cranial suspensory ligament. It is also attached to the gubernaculum testis, a jelly-like ligament that connects the testis and epididymis to the scrotum. The action of androgens causes this ligament to dissolve, and the action of growth factors causes the gubernaculum to contract. The combined effect is that the testis is drawn into the lower abdomen adjacent to the inguinal canal at around 12 weeks of gestation (B). Under the influence of androgens, the testis passes through the inguinal canal into the scrotum between 27 and 30 weeks of gestation (C).

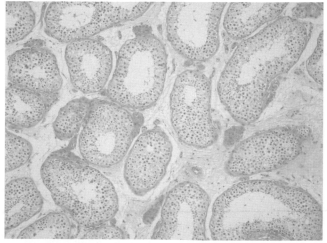

Fig. 6.3
Histological appearance of the testis. (Courtesy of Dr Dan Berney.)

functional part of the testis, the Leydig cells (or interstitial cells), lies between the seminiferous tubules (Fig. 6.4). The Leydig cells can function independently of the seminiferous tubules. However, the seminiferous tubules need functioning Leydig cells.

The seminiferous tubules consist of two cell types: Sertoli cells and germ cells (Fig. 6.5). At puberty there are around 600 million germ cells, called spermatogonia, per testis. The Sertoli cells provide both nutrition and hormonal support to allow the germ cells to develop into sperm, and functional Sertoli cells are required for spermatogenesis to occur. Each Sertoli cell is in contact with a number of germ cells. However, the relationship between the germ cells and Sertoli cells is not fully understood. The seminiferous tubules lead to the epididymis, where sperm maturation occurs.

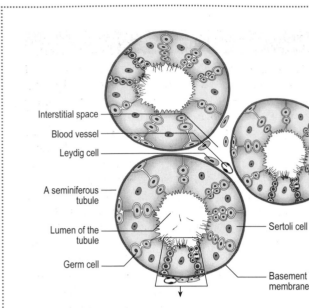

Fig. 6.4
Structure of the testes showing the arrangement of seminiferous tubules and a section through a seminiferous tubule. The area in the box is shown in more detail in Figure 6.5.

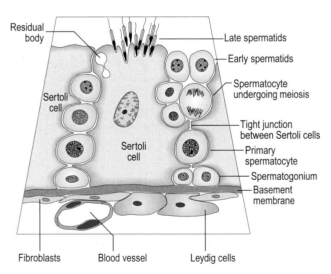

Fig. 6.5
Cells of the seminiferous tubule and the process of spermatogenesis. The germ cells originate next to the basement membrane, between the Sertoli cells. As these germ cells, known as spermatogonia, develop, they migrate towards the lumen of the seminiferous tubule, passing between the Sertoli cells. The immature spermatids are released from the secondary spermatogonia into the lumen of the seminiferous tubule, leaving 'residual bodies' behind. The spermatids mature into spermatozoa as they pass along the tubules and through the epididymis.

The epididymis is connected to the urethra by the vas deferens (see Fig. 6.1).

There is a blood–testis barrier, formed by the very tight contact between adjacent Sertoli cells. This barrier has an important role in maintaining an internal environment within the testis that is different from the blood or extracellular fluid. The intra-testicular fluid contains a testosterone binding protein which has an important role in maintaining a high intra-testicular testosterone concentration. It also functions to prevent fragments of immature sperm from entering the bloodstream and triggering an immune response: disruption of the blood–testis barrier has been proposed as the triggering event in the production of anti-sperm antibodies, resulting in sub-fertility. It is also thought that this barrier may protect sperm to some extent from blood-borne toxins.

Testicular blood supply

Blood supply to the testes is mainly through the testicular artery, which arises from the aorta. However, the testicular artery forms a network of connections with the internal iliac artery, which supplies the vas deferens, so that the blood supply to the testis effectively has two origins. Venous drainage is into the inferior vena cava on the right and the renal vein on the left. It is thought that the dual-origin blood supply may protect the testis from possible disruption. However, as the testis descends from the abdomen into the scrotum, it trails its blood vessels behind it. During the process of testicular descent, or at a later stage in life, the testis can twist, causing restriction of the blood supply or impaired venous drainage, which is treated as a surgical emergency.

Unexpected fracture box 1

Case history

John Smith, a 25-year-old man, came to the accident and emergency department after a fall. He had tripped while crossing the road and had fallen awkwardly. The main impact was on the right side of the chest. After the fall he had severe chest pain over the site of the impact.

The past medical history was unremarkable. Mr Smith was taking no medications and did not smoke or drink alcohol. He lived with his wife and worked as a chef. The couple had been attempting to have a baby for 2 years, with no success.

The examination showed him to be tall with long arms and legs. There was swelling of breast tissue underlying the nipple on both sides. The doctor found the right lower ribs to be very tender and there was bruising over the skin. There was scanty body, pubic and axillary hair, and the testes were very small (less than 2 mL in volume; normal >20 mL).

Chest radiography revealed several fractures in the right lower ribs. The doctor was concerned about the severity of the fractures despite the relatively trivial fall. The doctor was also concerned about the other findings on clinical examination.

Spermatogenesis

Spermatogenesis is the process by which the germ cells in the seminiferous tubules develop into mature sperm (see Fig. 6.5). There are three distinct stages to this process: proliferation of the spermatogonia, reduction of the number of chromosomes (meiosis) and development of the mature sperm structure. The spermatogonia are not used up during this process: after the second division of each stem cell, three of the spermatogonia continue on the pathway of cell division that leads to the production of sperm, while the fourth remains as a stem cell and begins dividing again to produce more spermatogonia. A healthy man produces around 200 million sperm every day, from puberty to old age. This adds up to over a trillion sperm over a lifetime. The whole process, from the start of spermatogonium differentiation to the formation of a mature sperm, takes 70 days, with a further 12–21 days required for transport of the sperm through the epididymis to the ejaculatory duct. Each spermatogonium gives rise to a total of 64 sperm. Each ejaculate contains approximately 200 million sperm, with the volume of the ejaculate (usually around 3 mL) made up of fluids from the seminal vesicles and prostate gland.

Interesting fact

Vasectomy is an irreversible form of contraception. A vasectomy is performed by cutting both of the vas deferens (see Fig. 6.1) and tying the cut ends. This prevents sperm from entering the ejaculate. A man who has had a vasectomy is still able to maintain an erection and to produce ejaculate as normal, but as no sperm are able to get through the cut vas deferens he is effectively infertile. He still produces sperm but these are simply absorbed back into the body. One interesting effect of vasectomy is the appearance of antibodies against spermatozoa; this occurs in about half of all vasectomized men. It is not known why this occurs but it contributes to the problems associated with attempted reversal of the vasectomy procedure.

Androgen production

The Leydig cell produces androgens which, like all steroid hormones, are made from cholesterol (Fig. 6.6). Androgens are 19-carbon steroids which can be readily interconverted to oestrogens through the actions of an enzyme called aromatase (Fig. 6.7). A range of androgens is made in the body and, although most of these come from the testes, some are made in the adrenal cortex (see Chapter 4). The most potent and important of these androgens is testosterone, and by far the highest production of testosterone is in the testes. The testis is not a highly vascular tissue like the adrenal cortex, and the presence of the blood–testis barrier and a specific androgen binding protein in the interstitial fluid of the testis means that high concentrations of testosterone accumulate. These high local levels of testosterone in the testis are important for spermatogenesis.

Hormonal control of testicular function

Both spermatogenesis and androgen secretion are controlled by the hypothalamus and pituitary glands

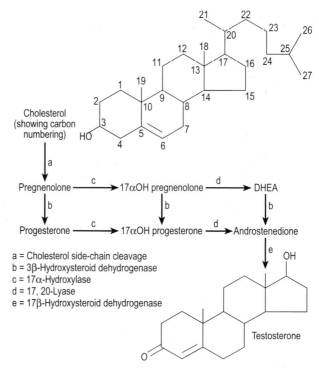

a = Cholesterol side-chain cleavage
b = 3β-Hydroxysteroid dehydrogenase
c = 17α-Hydroxylase
d = 17, 20-Lyase
e = 17β-Hydroxysteroid dehydrogenase

Fig. 6.6
Pathway of testosterone synthesis in Leydig cells. Cholesterol is the starting point for steroid biosynthesis in all steroid secreting tissues. The key shows all the enzyme activities involved in this biosynthetic pathway.

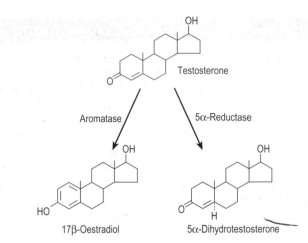

Fig. 6.7

Conversion of testosterone to 5α-dihydrotestosterone (DHT) and 17β-oestradiol. Testosterone itself is important for stimulating spermatogenesis but is converted to DHT in peripheral tissues to exert its classical hormonal effects. Testosterone is also converted to oestrogens, mainly 17β-oestradiol, by the actions of aromatase, an enzyme found in adipose tissues.

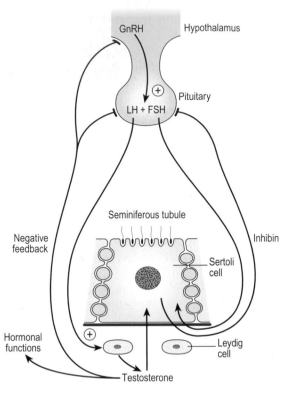

Fig. 6.8

Hypothalamo–pituitary–testis axis. Gonadotropin releasing hormone (GnRH), released from the hypothalamus, stimulates the gonadotroph cells of the anterior pituitary to release luteinizing hormone (LH) and follicle stimulating hormone (FSH). LH acts on Leydig cells to stimulate testosterone production, which acts with FSH on Sertoli cells to stimulate spermatogenesis. Testosterone and inhibin, a peptide secreted by Sertoli cells, exert negative feedback control of this axis.

(Fig. 6.8). The hypothalamic hormone, gonadotropin releasing hormone (GnRH), is secreted in a pulsatile manner to stimulate luteinizing hormone (LH) and follicle stimulating hormone (FSH) secretion. This pulsatile pattern of secretion is important: if GnRH is given as a constant infusion it actually inhibits secretion of these hormones. LH acts on the Leydig cells to stimulate testosterone synthesis, and the testosterone secreted by the Leydig cells acts together with FSH on the Sertoli cells to stimulate spermatogenesis (see Fig. 6.8). The process of spermatogenesis is absolutely dependent on the presence of an appropriate level of testosterone within the testis. However, although FSH stimulates Sertoli cell function it is not absolutely necessary for a low level of spermatogenesis to occur. Like LH (see Fig. 6.9), FSH binds to a G-protein-coupled receptor and stimulates adenylyl cyclase activity. However, a number of other pathways are also activated, including several kinase cascades. The action of testosterone on Sertoli cells appears to involve the opening of ligand-gated ion channels, in addition to the more usual transcriptional effects expected of a steroid.

There is negative feedback inhibition of the hypothalamo–pituitary–testicular axis, with testosterone inhibiting LH secretion. In addition, there are two peptide hormones secreted by the Sertoli cells that also have a role in regulating this axis: activin, which stimulates GnRH and FSH secretion, and inhibin, which inhibits FSH secretion. Inhibin may be used as a marker of Sertoli cell function as serum concentrations of this hormone are directly related to sperm count.

LH initiates testosterone synthesis by binding to receptors on the surface of Leydig cells. This generates cyclic adenosine monophosphate (cAMP) as a second messenger and initiates a series of reactions that lead to increased delivery of cholesterol to the mitochondrion, the rate-limiting step of steroidogenesis, as in the adrenal cortex (Fig. 6.9). In addition to stimulating spermatogenesis, FSH also causes the Sertoli cells to produce an androgen binding protein (ABP). This protein binds testosterone and helps maintain a high concentration of testosterone within the testes; this is essential for spermatogenesis to occur.

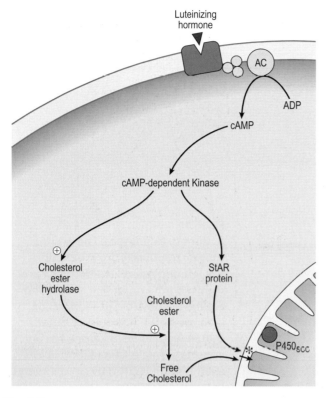

Fig. 6.9
Effects of luteinizing hormone (LH) on Leydig cells. Binding of LH to its receptor activates (via a G-protein, G_s) adenylyl cyclase (AC), which causes an increase in intracellular cyclic adenosine monophosphate (cAMP), resulting in activation of cAMP-dependent kinase. This phosphorylates and activates cholesterol ester hydrolase, liberating free cholesterol from intracellular pools, and also causes an increase in steroidogenic acute regulatory (StAR) protein. StAR protein facilitates the transport of cholesterol from the outer to the inner mitochondrial membrane (shown by an asterisk), allowing cholesterol access to the first enzyme of steroidogenesis: cholesterol side-chain cleavage ($P450_{scc}$). The rate of transfer of cholesterol from the outer to the inner mitochondrial membrane is what determines the rate of steroidogenesis – called the 'rate limiting step'.

Interesting fact

High concentrations of testosterone within the testes are required to support spermatogenesis, whereas only relatively low concentrations are needed to maintain potency (the ability to have and maintain an erection) and secondary sexual characteristics of men. This has been the basis of the development of a hormonal form of male contraceptive (see Chapter 8).

Transport of testosterone in blood

Testosterone is transported in blood bound to a carrier protein, called either testosterone binding globulin (TeBG) or, more commonly, sex hormone binding globulin (SHBG). In normal men, only about 2% of the circulating testosterone is unbound, with 44% bound to SHBG and 54% bound to serum albumin. The protein-bound testosterone is protected from metabolism in the liver and provides an easily accessible pool of hormone, as the testosterone readily dissociates from its binding protein. Levels of SHBG in plasma are regulated by androgens, oestrogens and thyroid hormones. In healthy men, SHBG levels are fairly constant, but may need to be considered when steroid replacement therapy is used.

Actions of testosterone

Testosterone has two main actions: the initiation of spermatogenesis and the development and maintenance of secondary sexual characteristics. In order to achieve the second group of actions, testosterone must be converted to 5α-dihydrotestosterone (DHT) (see Fig. 6.7). This conversion happens outside the testes, in peripheral tissues. Testosterone can also be converted to oestrogen by an enzyme called aromatase, which is found mainly in adipose tissue. Consequently, testosterone is sometimes described as a 'pre-hormone' or hormonal precursor, although this is not really correct as it is testosterone itself that acts to maintain spermatogenesis. In general, when the actions of testosterone are described, the effects of DHT are included in the description. The main physiological actions of testosterone and DHT are shown in Figure 6.10.

Testosterone is an anabolic androgenic steroid. As a steroid, testosterone acts on intracellular receptors to alter the rate of transcription of certain genes and thus increase the production of certain proteins.

Interesting fact

Because the enzyme aromatase is found mainly in adipose tissue, very obese men tend to convert more of their testosterone to oestrogen than lean men. This has feminizing effects, including breast development, decreased facial hair and altered pubic hair distribution.

In puberty, testosterone stimulates growth of long bones, causing an initial growth spurt, but then leads to fusing of the epiphyseal plates, resulting in cessation of long bone growth. Testosterone also causes

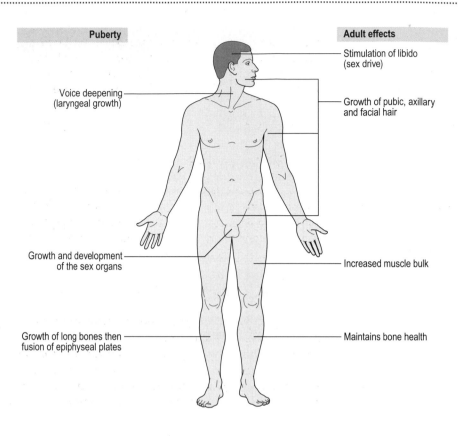

Puberty

Adult effects

Voice deepening
(laryngeal growth)

Growth and development
of the sex organs

Growth of long bones then
fusion of epiphyseal plates

Stimulation of libido
(sex drive)

Growth of pubic, axillary
and facial hair

Increased muscle bulk

Maintains bone health

Fig. 6.10
Actions of androgens. The actions specific to puberty are shown on the left and effects in adult men are shown on the right. The actions shown are mainly physiological effects on men. However, it should be noted that in women testosterone has an important role in stimulating libido, even though it circulates in only very low concentrations.

laryngeal growth, which results in deepening of the voice at puberty; this is pronounced in boys, but much less so in girls. In boys at puberty, testosterone causes growth of the penis, scrotum, prostate, seminal vesicles, epididymis and vas deferens.

In an adult man, testosterone is essential for the maintenance of secondary sexual characteristics. It enhances libido, is necessary for getting and maintaining an erection (potency), and stimulates the growth of facial and axillary hair. Testosterone is also necessary for bone health: testosterone deficiency causes osteoporosis. As an anabolic steroid, testosterone has a range of metabolic effects, acting to increase lean body mass and to alter plasma lipid composition. It also causes growth of skeletal muscle, an effect that is exploited by some athletes and body-builders (see below).

> ### Unexpected fracture box 2
>
> **Case note: Examination**
>
> Mr Smith had rib fractures after a small fall and this suggested that the underlying bones were not healthy. The most likely reason was osteoporosis due to a reduced level of sex steroids. The examination showed small testes, reduced body hair, increased

> breast tissue, and long arms and legs. These observations are all consistent with decreased androgen activity.
>
> Testosterone is required for male development and bone function. In Mr Smith's case, testosterone deficiency resulted in gynaecomastia, osteoporosis and reduced body hair. The long limbs are due to continuing growth due to delayed fusion of the growth plates, which is controlled by testosterone.

Disorders of male reproduction

Hypogonadism can arise through failure of testicular function (primary hypogonadism), pituitary failure (secondary hypogonadism) or, more rarely, hypothalamic failure (tertiary hypogonadism). Although the causes vary, the symptoms of hypogonadism experienced are common to all causes (Fig. 6.11).

Primary hypogonadism

This describes a disorder of testicular function itself, in the presence of normal hypothalamic and pituitary function. The most common cause of primary hypogonadism, also called hypergonadotropic hypogonadism, is Klinefelter's syndrome. Klinefelter's syndrome is a chromosomal abnormality that results in small testes

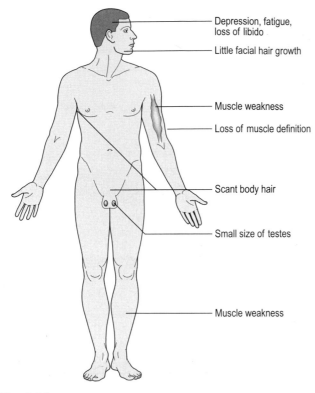

Depression, fatigue, loss of libido

Little facial hair growth

Muscle weakness

Loss of muscle definition

Scant body hair

Small size of testes

Muscle weakness

Fig. 6.11
Signs and symptoms of hypogonadism.

and failure of secondary sex characteristics. Other causes of primary hypogonadism include mumps orchitis, cryptorchidism (failure of testes to descend into scrotum) and testicular damage from radiation or chemotherapy.

Treatment of primary hypogonadism consists of steroid replacement therapy in order to maintain secondary sex characteristics – normal growth of pubic and axillary hair and sexual function. The infertility resulting from primary hypogonadism is not reversible.

Unexpected fracture box 2

Case note: Investigation

Blood tests revealed:

Luteinizing hormone (LH)	35 U/L (normal <10 U/L)
Follicle stimulating hormone (FSH)	65 U/L (normal <10 U/L)
Testosterone	4 nmol/L (normal 9–41 nmol/L)
Sperm count	Very low

The testis is controlled by LH and FSH. LH stimulates testosterone production from Leydig cells. FSH stimulates the Sertoli cells to initiate and then support

the maturation of germ cells into sperm. Mr Smith's results indicate that the testes were abnormal (this is called primary hypogonadism) and that both the Leydig cells and seminiferous tubules were not working.

Secondary hypogonadism

Also called hypogonadotropic hypogonadism, secondary hypogonadism is caused by failure of the pituitary gland to secrete appropriate quantities of the gonadotropins, LH and FSH. It is uncommon and usually associated with general hypopituitarism.

Tertiary hypogonadism

Tertiary hypogonadism, the other form of hypogonadotropic hypogonadism, is caused by failure of GnRH secretion from the hypothalamus. The most common cause of disordered GnRH secretion is Kallmann's syndrome, a hereditary disorder that is often associated with anosmia, an impaired sense of smell.

Unexpected fracture box 3

Case note: Diagnosis and treatment

The underlying reason for these findings was Klinefelter's syndrome. This is a common chromosomal abnormality with an incidence of 1 in 500 births. It involves a duplication of the X chromosome resulting in the abnormal karyotype 47XXY.

There is no cure for Klinefelter's syndrome. Mr Smith was infertile for life. However, testosterone replacement was given to improve bone and male development, and to prevent fractures.

Interesting fact

Some patients with Klinefelter's syndrome are chromosomal mosaics; in other words, their body cells are one of two different karyotypes (e.g. 46XY/47XXY). Chromosomal mosaics arise during cell division in a fertilized ovum and the result is a baby made up of two different cell lines. These cell lines can be randomly distributed in tissues (hence mosaic) or may result in some tissues being made up of normal cells and other tissues made of abnormal cells. In a Klinefelter mosaic, many of the gonadal cells will be abnormal (47XXY), resulting in low testosterone production.

Abuse of anabolic androgenic steroids

Testosterone replacement therapy is routinely given to treat the symptoms of hypogonadism, as in the case of Mr Smith. In such situations testosterone is very helpful in maintaining a normal masculine appearance and in preserving bone health. When testosterone is used in this way there are usually no problems with adverse effects. However, the situation is very different when these steroids are taken for other reasons, usually at high doses (Fig. 6.12).

Anabolic androgenic steroids (AASs) are abused mainly by young men. They may be taken by teenagers who want to improve their body image, by bodybuilders to increase muscle mass, or by athletes in power sports who will gain an advantage from increased muscle mass, enhanced aggression and, it is believed, improved endurance and faster recovery from injury. Although it may be argued that testosterone is a 'natural substance', when used as a drug of abuse it has a number of serious side effects, and the synthetic analogues of testosterone, such as tetrahydrogestrinone (THG) and stanozolol, have similar adverse effects. It is simply not possible to separate the 'desirable' anabolic effects from the 'undesirable' androgenic actions of these steroids.

One of the major side effects of using steroids is infertility. Synthetic AASs act just like testosterone itself in exerting negative feedback on the hypothalamus and pituitary, inhibiting gonadotropin secretion. This means that the testes will shrink (atrophy) and stop producing both testosterone and sperm. Women who abuse AASs are likely to become masculinized, developing a deep voice and increased body hair (hirsutism), while ceasing menstruation. There are other serious side effects due to the usual route of administration of these steroids: most androgens are harmful to the liver if taken orally, resulting in a significant risk of liver cancer.

Declining sperm counts

In the second half of the 20th century a number of studies reported that there was a decline in the average sperm count of men in the developed world. There have also been studies in wildlife populations

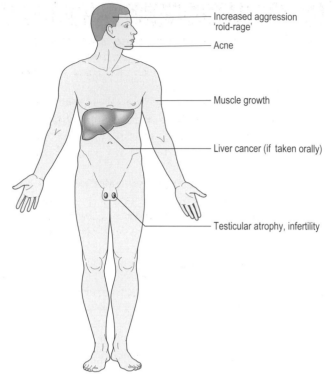

Fig. 6.12
Side effects of abusing anabolic androgenic steroids in men. In women there are additional problems, including the masculinizing effects of these steroids: deepening voice, facial hair growth, acquisition of male body shape, altered serum lipid profile and amenorrhoea.

reporting feminization of male fish, reptiles and some mammalian species, including a report on hermaphrodite polar bears. There is good evidence that the effects seen in wildlife populations are due to chemicals in the environment that have oestrogenic effects. These chemicals include pesticides, various organochlorides and excreted oestrogens in sewage effluent. They are properly classified as 'environmental endocrine disruptors' and have a wide range of effects on different endocrine systems. Almost inevitably, however, those chemicals with oestrogenic actions that cause feminization are termed 'gender benders'. Although the circumstantial evidence appears to be strong, there is presently no direct evidence that these chemicals are also responsible for the reported decline in human sperm counts.

Self-assessment case study

Mr Cheung, a 20-year-old man, presented with sweats and low mood. The symptoms began insidiously several months after treatment for a germ cell tumour and had been worsening for 6 months.

The tumour was discovered after he noticed a lump in the right testicle, and investigations and biopsy led to a diagnosis of a testicular seminoma. Six cycles of chemotherapy were performed and he had been declared in remission.

On examination now, he looked well. There was no fever. There was resolving alopecia and the remainder of the examination was normal, except the testes were 10 mL in volume. There were no testicular masses palpable.

Investigations showed:

Free T4	13.5 pmol/L (normal 9–22 pmol/L)
TSH	2.1 mU/L (normal 0.5–5 mU/L)
Testosterone	2.3 nmol/L (normal 9–35 nmol/L)
LH/FSH	23/31 U/L (normal <10 U/L)

Questions:

① What is the mechanism for the raised LH and FSH?

② What is the diagnosis?

③ What are the long-term risks and benefits of testosterone replacement?

Answers see page 148

Extended matching questions

A   Activin
B   Androgen binding protein (ABP)
C   Androstenedione
D   Dihydrotestosterone
E   Follicle stimulating hormone (FSH)
F   Gonadotropin releasing hormone (GnRH)
G   Inhibin
H   Luteinizing hormone (LH)
I   Sex hormone binding globulin (SHBG)
J   Stanozolol
K   Steroidogenic acute regulatory (StAR) protein
L   Testosterone

For each of the definitions below, select the appropriate substance from the list above:

① This acts on the Leydig cells to stimulate testosterone synthesis and secretion.

② This Sertoli cell product stimulates GnRH and FSH secretion.

③ This Sertoli cell product helps maintain high levels of testosterone within the testis.

④ This can be converted to oestradiol by the action of aromatase.

⑤ This is used as a marker of Sertoli cell function as blood levels are directly related to sperm count.

⑥ This synthetic androgen is anabolic and may be abused by athletes.

Answers see page 151

HORMONAL CONTROL OF REPRODUCTION PART II: FEMALE REPRODUCTIVE SYSTEM

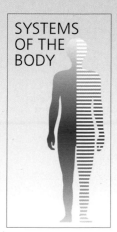

SYSTEMS OF THE BODY

Chapter objectives

After reading this chapter you should be able to:

① Describe the structure and function of the ovary and outline its relation to the other female reproductive organs.

② Describe the hormone secretion by the ovary and outline the functions of these hormones.

③ Describe the hormonal control of the menstrual cycle.

④ Outline the major hormonal disorders of the female reproductive system.

⑤ Explain the hormonal changes that occur in pregnancy.

⑥ Outline the hormonal control of parturition and lactation.

Introduction

There are some clear similarities between the male and female reproductive systems, but some very obvious differences. In men there is a relatively constant production of gametes both on a day-to-day basis and throughout adult life, whereas in women there is the production of a single egg each month, which ceases at about the age of 50 years. Although both male and female reproduction is regulated by the same hormones, it is clear that these need to act very differently to co-ordinate reproductive function in men and women.

Imbalanced sex steroids box 1

Case history

Joanna Jones was a 24-year-old woman who presented with increased facial and body hair, acne and irregular periods. The symptoms began when she was about 15 or 16 years old. She noticed coarse hair developing on her cheeks, under her chin, on the front of her chest and around her nipples. Acne appeared on her face and back, and her skin became greasy. Her periods began at the age of 11 years and were always unpredictable, but from age 15 years she noticed that she would miss one or two periods every 3 months.

Ms Jones' past medical history was unremarkable. She was taking no medications, cigarettes or alcohol. She was a shop assistant and lived with her parents. She had a boyfriend and the couple were planning marriage in the next 12 months and hoped to start a family.

The mother and a maternal aunt had type 2 diabetes mellitus.

On examination she weighed 85 kg and had a height of 163 cm, with body mass index of 32 kg/m^2. There was hirsutism over her face, chest, and on her lower body extending from the pubic region to the umbilicus. Her skin was greasy and marked by acne. Fundoscopy, visual fields and eye movements were normal.

① What is the differential diagnosis?

② Which tests should be performed to confirm the diagnosis?

③ How will her symptoms and tests guide treatment?

④ Will the couple be infertile?

Structure of the ovary

The ovaries are the female gonads. They have two main functions: the production of oocytes for fertilization, and the synthesis of female sex hormones – oestrogens and progestogens. There are two ovaries, lying in the abdomen on either side of the uterus. They are almond-shaped glands, approximately 4 cm long, and are connected to the uterus via the fallopian tubes (Fig. 7.1). The blood supply to the ovaries is from the ovarian arteries which arise directly from the aorta, just beneath the renal arteries. Venous drainage on the right is into the inferior vena cava, and on the left is into the renal vein. This is exactly the same as the venous drainage of the testes.

The ovary contains a number of follicles (Fig. 7.2). The great majority are primordial follicles, the pool of undeveloped oocytes. Unlike the system of gamete production in the male, which is a continuous process throughout life, a woman has only the number of oocytes she is born with, which develop and mature, usually one at a time, during her reproductive life. Typically there are millions of primordial follicles in the fetal ovary, with about 400 000 at the time of menarche (onset of menstrual bleeding).

Structurally, each primary oocyte is surrounded by a single layer of granulosa cells within a basement membrane. During the reproductive life of a woman, between puberty and menopause, many of these primordial follicles will grow to form mature oocytes, one of which is released at ovulation each month. The development of a primordial follicle into a mature oocyte (Fig. 7.3) takes several months and starts with

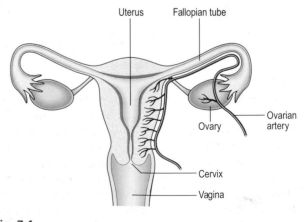

Fig. 7.1
The female reproductive system.

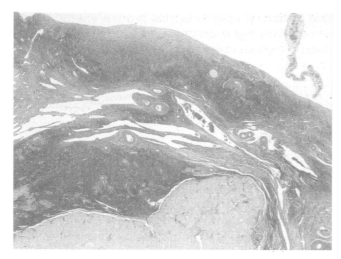

Fig. 7.2
Histology of the ovary. (Courtesy of Dr Daniel Berney.)

the process of follicle recruitment: the selection of one primordial follicle for further development. This process is known to be independent of the gonadotropins; recent evidence has implicated the anti-mullerian hormone (see Chapter 8) as an inhibitor of follicular response to FSH, but otherwise little is understood about the process of follicle selection.

As the primordial follicle develops, the single layer of cells around it divides and forms the granulosa cell layer (see Fig. 7.3). As the follicle develops further, stromal cells grow around the outside of the follicle to form the theca layer. After ovulation these granulosa and theca cells remain actively secretory and comprise the corpus luteum 'yellow body', although immediately after ovulation the ruptured follicle fills with blood and appears as a red haemorrhagic body in the ovary. The corpus luteum gradually regresses

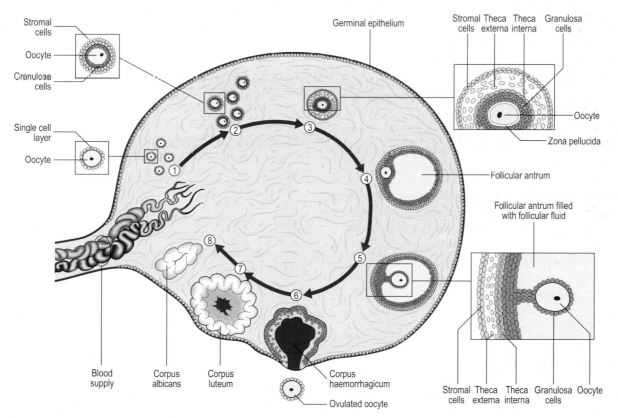

Fig. 7.3
Stages of follicular development in the ovary. (1) Primordial follicles consist of an oocyte surrounded by a single cell layer. (2) At the start of follicular development the cells divide to form a stromal layer and surround the granulosa cells. (3) Follicular development continues with the formation of the theca cells, which lie between the granulosa and stromal cells. The oocyte is surrounded by the zona pellucida. (4) The follicular antrum develops, filled with follicular fluid. (5) A mature oocyte: suspended in the follicular fluid, attached by a stalk to the granulosa cell layer. (6) As the follicle ruptures to release the oocyte (the point of ovulation), the antrum fills with blood to form a corpus haemorrhagicum, which develops into the corpus luteum (7). Regression of the corpus luteum leads to the formation of the scar-like corpus albicans (8). The whole cycle shown here takes several months. The developing follicles are not drawn to scale; for comparison, the follicle at stage 2 is around $20\,\mu m$ in diameter whereas the mature follicle at stage 5 is 250 times larger at 5 mm, easily visible by eye.

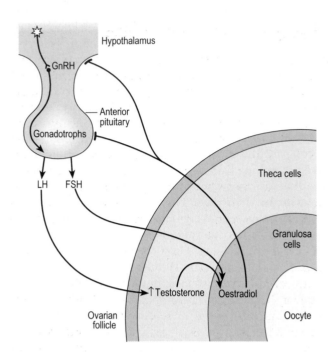

Fig. 7.4

Hormonal control of steroidogenesis in the ovarian follicle. The pulsatile release of gonadotropin releasing hormone (GnRH) from the hypothalamus stimulates release of luteinizing hormone (LH) and follicle stimulating hormone (FSH) from the gonadotroph cells of the anterior pituitary. LH receptors are located on the theca cells and LH binds to these receptors, stimulating the secretion of androgens, particularly testosterone. The testosterone is converted to oestradiol in granulosa cells. Levels of the enzyme that catalyses this reaction, aromatase, are increased by the action of FSH on the granulosa cells. Oestradiol exerts a negative feedback effect on the hypothalamus and pituitary.

by a process of apoptosis (this process was originally identified in the ovary) to form a scar-like enclosure called the corpus albicans (see Fig. 7.3).

Ovarian hormones

The function of the ovary is twofold: the production of oocytes and the secretion of hormones. The hormones secreted include the steroids (oestrogens, progesterone and androgens) and the peptides (inhibin, activin and relaxin). Oestrogens and progesterone have an important role in maintaining the endometrial lining of the uterus (see The menstrual cycle below) and in negative feedback regulation of pituitary hormone release (Fig. 7.4). In contrast to the steroid hormones, the ovarian peptide hormones were discovered more recently and their functions are less well understood. These steroid and peptide hormones are secreted by the cells of the developing follicle, the theca cells and the granulosa cells (see Fig. 7.3), as well as by the corpus luteum.

Oestrogens

The ovaries secrete a range of oestrogens, the female sex steroids, with the principal and most potent of these being oestradiol (Fig. 7.5). There is a close functional interaction between the theca and granulosa cells in the ovary: the theca cells secrete androgens in response to luteinizing hormone (LH) stimulation and this is converted to oestrogens by the adjacent granulosa cells under follicle stimulating hormone (FSH) control. The ovaries also secrete oestrone and oestriol, although these are also made by conversion of circulating androgens in peripheral tissues.

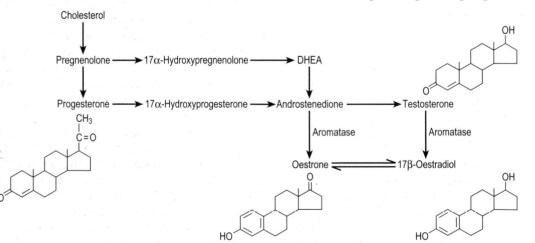

Fig. 7.5

Biosynthesis of the major ovarian steroids. Progesterone is both the major secretory product of the corpus luteum and an intermediate in the synthesis of other steroids. Testosterone is synthesized by the theca cells of the follicle and converted into oestradiol by the granulosa cells. DHEA, dehydroepiandrosterone.

The oestrogens are responsible for the development and maintenance of the secondary sexual characteristics of women, including breast development. They maintain the structure of the vaginal mucosa and stimulate cervical mucus production, maintaining vaginal lubrication. Oestrogens are very important for bone health, particularly during the pubertal period, and are thought to be protective against cardiovascular disease. Oestrogens also promote uterine development during the menstrual cycle (see below).

Interesting fact

Things are not always as straightforward as they seem. It was observed, some years back, that cows that grazed on fields sprayed with certain pesticides, such as DDT, had lowered fertility rates. The conclusion would seem to be that chemicals like DDT have toxic effects on cows' reproductive systems. However, some of the compounds produced by plants, particularly the isoflavenoids, have weak oestrogenic activity in animals. Plants use these 'phyto-oestrogens' for a variety of functions, including attracting beneficial bacteria to the plants' roots to aid growth. It turned out that chemicals like DDT reduced the plants' ability to attract these bacteria and, in an attempt to attract more, plants such as clover were producing greatly increased amounts of isoflavenoids. In sufficiently large quantities, the weak oestrogenic activity of the ingested flavenoids had a contraceptive effect on the cows, reducing overall fertility. This is a good example of the 'endocrine disruptor' effect of some environmental chemicals, opening up a whole new branch of endocrinology.

Progesterone

Progesterone is secreted principally by the corpus luteum. Several steroids have similar properties and are together classified as the 'progestogens'. These include 17α-hydroxyprogesterone and pregnenolone as well as progesterone itself (see Fig. 7.5). Progesterone is responsible for maintaining the structure of the uterus to allow implantation of the embryo, and has an essential role in the maintenance of pregnancy. It is a thermogenic steroid, acting to raise body temperature. This property may be exploited in determining a woman's fertile period each month, as there is a small but fairly reliable rise in body temperature as a result of increased progesterone secretion following ovulation (see Fig. 7.6D).

Androgen secretion by the ovaries

It may seem surprising to read that the ovary produces androgens, the classical male sex steroids, but these hormones have important functions in women. First, they are essential in the production of oestrogens: the enzyme aromatase converts androgens to oestrogens in both the ovary and adipose tissues (see Fig. 7.5). Second, androgens are responsible for the development and maintenance of pubic and axillary hair, and also have an important role in controlling sex drive (libido). The most potent androgen in women, as in men, is testosterone. Much of the circulating testosterone in women comes directly from the ovaries, but the rest is produced by conversion of adrenal androgens (see Chapter 4). The normal circulating concentration of testosterone in adult women is between 0.5 and 2.5 nmol/L, compared with a range of 9 to 35 nmol/L in men. However, the amount of bioavailable testosterone is considerably lower than this in women as they have higher levels of the plasma binding protein, sex hormone binding globulin (SHBG) than men. There are also less potent androgens produced by the ovaries and adrenal, such as androstenedione and dehydroepiandrosterone (DHEA), that contribute significantly to the total amount of circulating androgen. Excessive androgen production by the ovaries (or adrenals) causes a degree of masculinization and disruption of the normal menstrual cycle. This is described in more detail below in the section on polycystic ovarian syndrome.

Ovarian peptide hormones

Inhibin was coined as a term in the 1930s, but the peptide hormone was isolated only in the 1980s. It is a glycoprotein, secreted by the granulosa and theca cells of the developing follicle, and has a role in inhibiting FSH secretion. It has been suggested that inhibin may have a role in follicle selection. Inhibin levels may also be an early marker of the onset of menopause.

Activin is a member of the transforming growth factor-β (TGF-β) peptide family. It was also isolated in the 1980s as a potential reproductive hormone but is now thought to have a role in the inflammatory response. High concentrations of activin are also produced by the endometrium and have a role in the development of the endometrium during the menstrual cycle. Clinically, activin may have a role as a prognostic indicator in women undergoing treatment to stimulate ovulation, as part of assisted conception.

Relaxin was first identified in the 1920s. It is now known that there are seven members of the relaxin family of peptides, with a range of different roles.

Relaxin stimulates follicular development and oocyte maturation, and may have a role in implantation of the embryo. It is known to have an important role in parturition and has a number of other effects outside the reproduction system, including an antifibrotic action in wound healing.

Transport of ovarian hormones in blood

Oestrogens are transported bound to sex hormone binding globulin (SHBG), a plasma protein. The concentration of SHBG in blood is regulated by steroid hormones, being increased by oestrogen and decreased by testosterone. Women therefore have around twice as much SHBG in their blood as men. Progesterone, on the other hand, does not have a specific plasma transport protein and is mostly carried in blood loosely bound to albumin.

Imbalanced sex steroids box 2

Case note: Differential diagnosis

Joanna's symptoms suggest a disruption of the sex steroid endocrinology. Such diseases can be classified into: excess male hormones or reduced female hormones.

The causes of reduced female hormones can be further separated into diseases of the pituitary/hypothalamus or ovarian failure. There were no symptoms or signs of pituitary or hypothalamic disease (for example, a visual field defect) or of ovarian failure (for example, flushing).

The symptoms suggested an excess of male hormones. The commonest cause of this is polycystic ovary syndrome. Rare causes include androgen secreting ovarian or adrenal tumours, or the genetic condition congenital adrenal hyperplasia (see Chapter 4). For every 100 patients with Joanna's symptoms, 98 will have polycystic ovary syndrome and only 2% will suffer from one of the other conditions.

Which tests would you perform to confirm the diagnosis?

Hormonal regulation of ovarian function

Ovarian function is controlled by the two gonadotropins, luteinizing hormone (LH) and follicle stimulating hormone (FSH), secreted by the gonadotrope cells of the anterior pituitary under the control of gonadotropin releasing hormone (GnRH) from the hypothalamus

(see Fig. 7.4). Release of these hormones is pulsatile, with both the amplitude and the frequency of pulses varying through the menstrual cycle.

The basic principle of the hormonal control of ovarian function is simple. The hormones do what their names suggest: FSH stimulates the growth of the developing follicle, and LH stimulates steroid production by the corpus luteum and the developing follicle. A surge in the production of LH is responsible for stimulating ovulation. There is only one small complication: although LH stimulates androgen secretion by the follicle, it is under the control of FSH that this is converted to oestrogen.

The menstrual cycle

This is the term given to the cycle of hormonal and other physiological changes that commences with the shedding of the endometrium (the uterine lining) and includes the release of a mature oocyte from the ovarian follicle. It is the basic unit of reproduction in women, producing a single mature germ cell each month, and is essential for understanding the reproductive process (Fig. 7.6). The average menstrual cycle lasts for 28 days – hence the term 'menstrual', meaning 'monthly'. Cycle length is usually fairly regular for an individual, but can vary between women over a considerable range, with most women having a cycle between 21 and 35 days long. In puberty and in the peri-menopausal period the cycle length may be considerably longer. The variation in cycle length is almost always due to variations in the follicular/proliferative phase.

There are several phases to the menstrual cycle that describe changes to both the ovary and the uterus.

The menstrual phase

In most numbering conventions, day 1 of the menstrual cycle is the day on which endometrial shedding starts. For a woman it is the first day of her monthly 'period'. The endometrial lining of the uterus, which has developed during the previous cycle, is shed through the vagina together with a small amount of blood. This vaginal bleeding usually lasts between 4 and 7 days. There are several disorders associated with menstruation, with perhaps the commonest being *dysmenorrhoea*, a term applied to the painful abdominal cramps experienced by many women during their period. This vasospasm is probably due to the high levels of prostaglandin production by the endometrium.

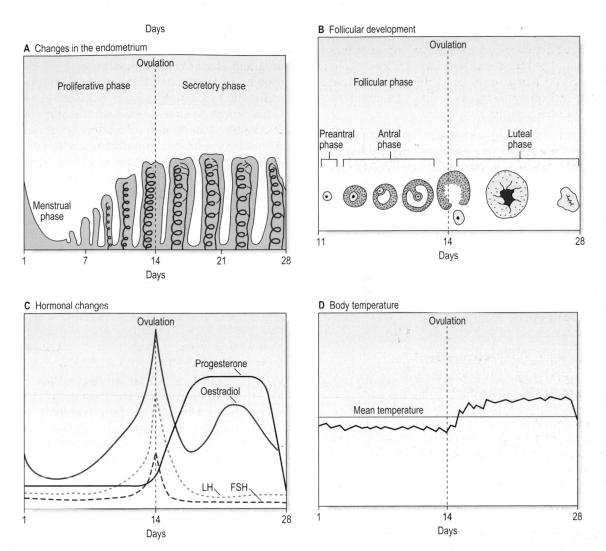

Fig. 7.6
The menstrual cycle. Conventionally the days of the menstrual cycle are numbered from the onset of menstruation (day 1). Ovulation occurs on day 14 in the standard 28-day cycle. The duration of the proliferative phase (the interval from the onset of menstruation to ovulation) is variable and ovulation does not always occur on day 14. However, there is little variation in the length of the secretory phase. (A) Changes in the endometrium during the menstrual cycle. (B) Stages of follicular development during the menstrual cycle. (C) Hormonal changes during the menstrual cycle; the peak in oestradiol immediately precedes ovulation. (D) Changes in body temperature during the menstrual cycle. Basal body temperature rises, under the influence of progesterone, after ovulation and remains higher than mean during the secretory phase, falling to slightly below mean temperature with the onset of menstruation.

The follicular phase (also called the proliferative phase)

The follicular phase of the cycle is dominated by oestrogen action. During this phase, the selected follicle undergoes the last stages of its maturation within the ovary prior to release of the oocyte. Gonadotropin secretion from the pituitary stimulates oestrogen synthesis by the developing follicle. Usually, increasing oestrogen levels would inhibit further gonadotropin release, but this negative feedback mechanism is suspended during the late follicular phase, and there is a peak in LH secretion which immediately precedes ovulation (see Fig. 7.6).

The proliferative phase describes the changes that occur in the uterus while the follicle is maturing in the ovary, prior to ovulation. Under the influence of oestrogens secreted by the follicle before ovulation, the endometrium proliferates and develops a rich blood supply. This process is called 'decidualization' of the endometrium. After ovulation takes place, the growth of the endometrium is maintained primarily by the progesterone secreted by the corpus luteum (see below).

The luteal phase (also called the secretory phase)

The luteal phase is dominated by the actions of progesterone. After ovulation the ruptured follicle from which the ovum was released forms a corpus luteum. This structure has a limited life of around 14 days, unless the ovum is fertilized, in which case the corpus luteum persists. In the absence of a fertilized ovum the corpus luteum degenerates – a process termed 'luteolysis' – and stops secreting progesterone. It is this decrease in progesterone secretion that causes the breakdown of the endometrium and the start of menstruation.

The luteal phase is also referred to as the 'secretory phase'. This refers both to the secretion of progesterone from the corpus luteum and to the secretion of a clear fluid by the endometrium during this phase.

Interesting fact

Only higher primates have menstrual cycles with regular bleeding. Lower mammals have an oestrous cycle that does not include menstruation; instead the uterine lining is broken down and resorbed. The oestrous cycle is most easily understood as a cycle of sexual receptivity. The word 'oestrous' comes from the Greek for the gadfly, suggesting the frenzied activity exhibited by some mammals when 'in heat'. Many mammals are 'continuous cyclers', like humans, whereas others have seasonal oestrous cycles with only one (cows and pigs) or two (dogs) cycles per year.

Imbalanced sex steroids box 3

Case note: Investigations

Joanna had a morning blood sample taken on day 21 of her menstrual cycle and an ultrasonographic scan of the ovaries was performed.

Prolactin	365 mU/L (normal <400 mU/L)
LH/FSH	18/4 U/L (normal <10 U/L)
Oestradiol	639 pmol/L (normal luteal phase 400–1200 pmol/L)
Progesterone	<3 nmol/L (normal luteal phase >30 nmol/L)
Cortisol	314 nmol/L (normal 200–600 nmol/L)
Testosterone	2.1 nmol/L (normal <3 nmol/L)
SHBG	25 nmol/L (normal 20–120 nmol/L)
Androstenedione	17.2 nmol/L (normal <8 nmol/L)
Dehydroepiandrosterone sulphate (DHEAS)	6.1 μmol/L (normal <6.8 μmol/L)
17α-Hydroxyprogesterone	3.7 nmol/L (normal <10 nmol/L)
Ultrasonography	Multiple cysts in both ovaries with increased stroma between the cysts.

The prolactin and oestradiol levels were normal, which made a pituitary or hypothalamic cause for her disease unlikely. The normal 17α-hydroxyprogesterone concentration made congenital adrenal hyperplasia less likely.

Virilizing adrenal or ovarian tumours often produce high serum testosterone levels (frequently >5 nmol/L), making these diagnoses less likely. Cushing's syndrome is due to an excess of cortisol, and adrenal production of androgens may also be increased. Thus, Cushing's syndrome may cause similar symptoms (but usually gives a thin skin rather than a thick skin). Here, the normal serum cortisol level made this diagnosis less likely.

These results are common for polycystic ovary syndrome. The male hormones are either high (androstenedione) or in the upper part of the normal range (testosterone and DHEAS), and the SHBG concentration is low. SHBG circulates with testosterone and inactivates it. A low serum SHBG level exacerbates the imbalance of male hormones. The LH/FSH ratio is characteristically higher in polycystic ovary syndrome, for unknown reasons.

The ultrasonographic appearances supported the diagnosis. However, ultrasonography of the ovaries is not a reliable diagnostic tool in polycystic ovary syndrome. This is because about 20% of healthy women with no symptoms of endocrine disease show multiple cysts on ultrasonography and do not have polycystic ovary syndrome.

The cause of polycystic ovary syndrome is unknown, but it is linked to increased body weight, insulin resistance (presumably causing a thickened skin) and a risk of diabetes mellitus. The working definition of polycystic ovary syndrome is the presence of symptoms of androgen excess with raised serum androgen levels *and* the exclusion of other diseases.

How will Joanna's symptoms and test results guide treatment?

Disorders of the menstrual cycle

Amenorrhoea is either the absence of menarche in a girl by the age of 16 years, or the failure of three or more menstrual periods in succession in a woman who previously had an established cycle. There are many causes of amenorrhoea, but the commonest by far is pregnancy. The first investigation to be carried out in a woman who presents with amenorrhoea should always be a pregnancy test. Other causes of amenorrhoea can be broadly divided into primary (ovarian failure), secondary (pituitary failure) and tertiary (hypothalamic failure), although amenorrhoea may also result from other endocrine disorders such as adrenal disorders. We shall start by looking at the hypothalamus.

Hypothalamic causes

This is one of the commonest causes of non-pregnant amenorrhoea, and is the underlying problem in about a third of cases. Hypothalamic causes include the amenorrhoea associated with excessive exercise and with eating disorders. In these disorders there is severe disruption of the hypothalamic secretion of GnRH, which leads to failure of pituitary LH and FSH secretion, and then to impaired ovarian function. It is likely that a decrease in body mass and in the proportion of body fat may contribute to the impaired GnRH secretion, and it is thought that leptin may be the link between body fat and hypothalamic function (see Chapter 11).

Pituitary causes

Hyperprolactinaemia accounts for approximately one-third of cases of non-pregnant amenorrhoea. It has been suggested that up to 5% of the adult population have an undiagnosed pituitary micro-prolactinoma, producing excessive amounts of prolactin. Prolactin is well known to cause disturbances of the menstrual cycle because it inhibits the pulsatile secretion of hypothalamic GnRH. In lactating women the high levels of circulating prolactin can be a useful, although not totally reliable, form of contraception. Hyperprolactinaemia is treated with bromocriptine, a dopamine antagonist.

Any disorder causing functional disturbance of anterior pituitary function will result in impaired gonadotropin secretion (see Chapter 3).

Ovarian causes

Premature ovarian failure

Ovarian failure at the appropriate time is called menopause and will be considered in the next chapter. Premature ovarian failure, which is also called premature menopause, is diagnosed when ovarian failure occurs before the age of 40 years. This is not a common disorder. There is often a genetic cause, such as Turner's syndrome, which is characterized by the absence of one X chromosome. It occurs in around 1 in 3000 female babies. Other causes include autoimmune destruction of the ovary, which is usually associated with other autoimmune disease, such as Graves' disease.

Polycystic ovarian syndrome (PCOS)

This syndrome is a common cause of amenorrhoea, accounting for up to 20% of cases. It is characterized by excessive androgen secretion, which is not a result of congenital adrenal hyperplasia or other cause. The excessive androgen secretion is often the problem that causes the patient to visit her doctor. She may notice increased facial and body hair, greasy skin and acne as well as irregular monthly periods (Fig. 7.7). Ultrasonographic examination of the ovaries reveals enlarged ovaries containing numerous cysts, from 2 to 8 mm in size. However, ovarian cysts are very common and may be present in 20% of women who have no menstrual irregularity and who do not have PCOS. PCOS cannot be seen as a purely ovarian disorder: type 2 diabetes mellitus is a common finding in women with PCOS and 50% of women with PCOS are clinically obese. Although women with PCOS usually

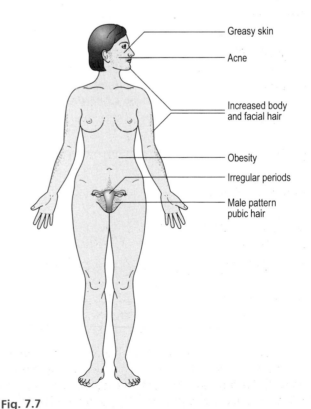

Fig. 7.7
Common features of polycystic ovarian syndrome (PCOS).

experience menstrual irregularities and thus reduced fertility, many still ovulate occasionally. There is a great variation between individuals in the degree of reduced fertility caused by PCOS.

The treatment for this disorder is generally just to manage the symptoms, as there is no cure at present. The mainline treatment is to use synthetic oestrogens and progestogens (as in the contraceptive pill) to reduce LH and FSH secretion and ovarian steroid secretion. This has the effect of decreasing the amount of androgen produced and so of reversing the effects of excessive androgen secretion. In some cases an androgen receptor antagonist can be used too.

Interesting fact

Some years ago a lot of interest was aroused by studies that seemed to show that groups of women living together, for example at boarding school, in religious institutions or in prisons, tended to have synchronized menstrual cycles. Subsequent studies have not supported this idea and have shown that, generally, synchronization does not occur in women, although there is good evidence for it in other species. Despite this, there has been an increased interest in the proposed mechanism of synchronization: pheromones. A pheromone is a chemical signal produced by one individual that causes behavioural changes in another without consciously being detected by the senses. Pheromones are therefore quite different from scents, which are detected by the olfactory apparatus. It has been known for some time that pheromones are important modulators of animal behaviour, but there is increasing evidence that there are also human pheromones. Their role remains a matter of speculation.

Imbalanced sex steroids box 4

Case note: Treatment

How will Joanna Jones' symptoms, test results and future plans guide treatment? There is no cure for polycystic ovary syndrome, because the cause is unknown. It is not even clear that the ovaries are the sole source of the increased levels of androgens. Adrenal and ovarian vein catheter studies have shown androgen production from both the ovaries and the adrenal glands. This makes surgical treatment unrealistic. Nearly all patients find hirsutism and acne very distressing. These problems can be

controlled with a combination of drugs: oestradiol to counterbalance the androgens, and an androgen blocker or inhibitor to lower the effect of the androgens on the skin. However, the couple desire a family and this combination of treatments will act as an oral contraceptive and may harm sexual development in a male fetus. So, if pregnancy is the main goal, other treatments will be needed.

Imbalanced sex steroids box 5

Case note: Fertility

Will the couple be infertile? Joanna was not ovulating regularly, as her menstrual cycle was not regular and the progesterone level taken on day 21 of the cycle was undetectable, indicating an infertile cycle. So it is likely that Joanna will have reduced fertility. However, fertility is difficult to predict as some patients with severe polycystic ovary syndrome still ovulate intermittently. Thus, if the couple do not desire pregnancy, they should be advised to use contraception.

In order to induce ovulation, Joanna will need a diet and exercise programme to improve her weight and insulin resistance. The drug metformin lowers insulin resistance (see Chapter 9) and may improve ovulation. Clomifene (a partial oestrogen receptor agonist) is effective when used together with metformin in stimulating ovulation. It is likely that the couple will be able to conceive with treatment.

The endocrinology of pregnancy

The placenta as an endocrine organ

When the released ovum is fertilized by a spermatozoon, then pregnancy results. Fertilization may occur in either the fallopian tubes or the uterus. The conceptus becomes embedded in the endometrial lining of the uterus and establishes a blood supply via the placenta. The placenta is also the major endocrine tissue of pregnancy. It sends hormonal signals to the corpus luteum, preventing luteal regression and maintaining progesterone and oestrogen secretion for the early part of pregnancy.

The major hormone produced by the placenta in the first weeks of gestation (pregnancy) is human chorionic gonadotropin (hCG) (see Fig. 7.10). hCG is structurally very similar to LH and has an important role in maintaining luteal function and preventing the

Box 7.1

Pregnancy testing

Detection of hCG is the basis of all pregnancy tests. As hCG is normally produced only during pregnancy it is a reliable and specific indicator of pregnancy. Although it is a fairly large peptide hormone, sufficient hCG is excreted in urine to be detectable by a variety of methods.

Old-fashioned pregnancy testing (Fig. 7.8)

The first pregnancy tests were bioassays for hCG. At first mice were used: groups of five immature female mice were injected with urine then killed some days later. Their ovaries and uterus were inspected, with 'enlargement' confirming the pregnancy. This used large numbers of mice and was fairly unreliable.

In the mid 20th century (1930s to 1960s) a simpler bioassay was developed. This was based on the observation that the female *Xenopus* toad (*Xenopus laevis*) would ovulate within 12 hours after exposure to hCG. Colonies of these toads were kept in pregnancy testing laboratories, injected with urine samples and checked for ovulation. Ovulation is not easy to miss in a *Xenopus* toad. This test was nearly 100% reliable, the results were available the next day, and the method had the advantage of re-usable toads. It did take a lot of worms, however, to keep the colonies going.

Modern pregnancy testing kit (Fig. 7.9)

The *Xenopus* colonies gradually fell into disuse as more sophisticated immunoassay methods were developed. Modern pregnancy testing kits use a sensitive immunoassay which can detect hCG from about 10 days after conception. The assay uses a colour-change reaction to indicate whether hCG is detected or not. The great advantage of this method is that it can be carried out conveniently at home.

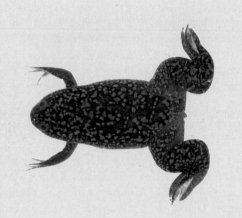

Fig. 7.8
Female *Xenopus* toad (*Xenopus laevis*), used in pregnancy tests. (Courtesy of and reproduced with permission of Xenbase.org.)

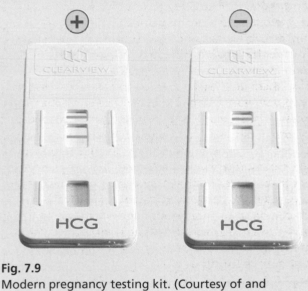

Fig. 7.9
Modern pregnancy testing kit. (Courtesy of and reproduced with permission of Unipath.)

normal regression of the corpus luteum, which ends an infertile menstrual cycle. Box 7.1 outlines how methods of detecting hCG have been developed over the years in pregnancy testing.

The placenta also produces steroids, and after about 8 weeks' gestation takes over from the corpus luteum as the major source of progesterone. The placental secretion of progesterone increases throughout pregnancy and is essential to maintain pregnancy. It is thought that progesterone acts to keep the myometrium (the muscular lining of the uterus) in a relaxed state, preventing contractions and expulsion of the fetus. This is partly achieved by inhibiting oxytocin receptor expression. Progesterone may also have a role in appetite and energy regulation.

Other steroids produced by the placenta include the oestrogens, oestrone, oestradiol and oestriol, levels of which all increase throughout pregnancy (Fig. 7.10). The placenta also secretes testosterone, which increases in concentration during pregnancy, reaching 10 times pre-pregnancy levels at term, as well as a placental lactogen (hPL), which stimulates breast development. hPL is closely related to growth hormone and prolactin, and also acts to antagonize

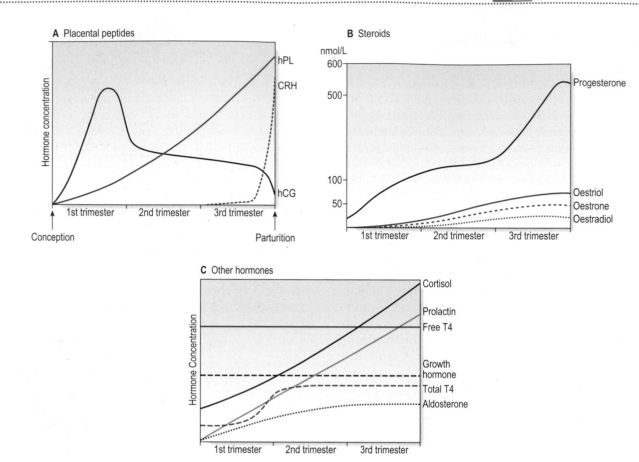

Fig. 7.10

Changes in the plasma concentrations of different hormones during pregnancy. (A) Placental peptides. Human chorionic gonadotropin (hCG) is the major peptide secreted in the first trimester, and peaks at around 10 weeks of gestation. Levels of human placental lactogen (hPL), in contrast, rise gradually throughout gestation, peaking just before parturition. Corticotropin releasing hormone (CRH) is the third placental peptide, and is a hormone of late pregnancy, increasing only about 3 weeks before parturition. (B) Steroid hormones. Progesterone is the major steroid hormone of pregnancy, with levels increasing throughout gestation, peaking just before parturition and falling sharply afterwards. Of the other steroids, oestriol is the major oestrogen. Levels of all the oestrogens rise gradually during pregnancy. Testosterone concentration, not shown here, also increases throughout pregnancy. (C) Other hormones. Levels of the adrenal hormones, cortisol and aldosterone, increase during pregnancy, with aldosterone reaching a plateau during the third trimester. Total thyroxine concentration increases during the first trimester, although there is no change in free T4 or free T3. Levels of prolactin, from the anterior pituitary, increase throughout pregnancy, but there is no change in growth hormone secretion.

the effects of insulin, which may have the effect of increasing the supply of nutrients to the fetus. The secretion of hPL increases throughout pregnancy.

Non-placental hormones in pregnancy

In addition to the hormones secreted by the placenta during pregnancy, there are other major effects on the endocrine system (see Fig. 7.10). Thyroid hormone secretion increases during the first trimester of pregnancy and then reaches a plateau, although thyroid hormone binding globulin (THBG) concentration increases as well, so there is no overall change in free thyroxine levels. Cortisol secretion increases throughout pregnancy, reaching three times the pre-pregnancy level at term, although adrenocorticotropic hormone (ACTH) secretion is unchanged. From the anterior pituitary, LH and FSH levels are very low throughout pregnancy, while the level of thyroid stimulating hormone (TSH) dips during the first trimester and then returns to pre-pregnancy levels. Growth hormone secretion is unchanged, but prolactin levels rise progressively throughout pregnancy.

Endocrine control of parturition

The signals that initiate parturition (labour) in humans are not well understood. Several hormones are known to be involved, including corticotropin releasing hormone (CRH), which is secreted by the placenta from about 20 days before parturition starts. A decline in progesterone concentration is also involved, as parturition can be initiated by giving the progesterone antagonist RU486. The ovarian peptide hormone, relaxin, has an important role in parturition, promoting cervical ripening. This is the process of growth and softening of the cervix, allowing delivery of the fetus.

In hospital, labour can be induced artificially by the administration of vaginal prostaglandins and injections of oxytocin. However, an increase in oxytocin concentration does not usually occur before the onset of parturition and so does not appear normally to be responsible for initiating labour. Oxytocin is probably more important for co-ordinating contraction of the myometrium, as levels rise rapidly *during* parturition. Prostaglandins are an important part of the onset of labour as they cause 'ripening' and dilation of the cervix.

It is now thought that the most important signal for labour to start is the increase in corticotropin releasing hormone (CRH) activity in the late stages of pregnancy. This rise is a signal for increased prostaglandin synthesis. However, the onset of parturition is more complex than an increase in the level of a single hormone, and it is clear that there is an interaction between many different hormonal signals.

Lactation

During pregnancy there is an interaction between several different hormones to stimulate breast development (Fig. 7.11). These include progesterone, human placental lactogen (hPL), prolactin, insulin and cortisol. However, the high oestrogen levels seen during pregnancy put a 'brake' on lactation. This brake is removed by delivery of the baby, which results in a rapid decrease of oestrogen levels and the onset of lactation, mostly under the control of prolactin. Suckling of the baby at the nipple stimulates the release of prolactin from the anterior pituitary and of oxytocin from

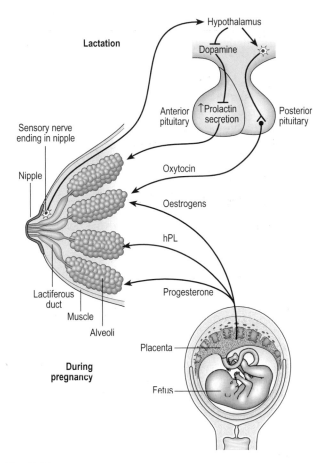

Fig. 7.11
Hormonal control of breast development during pregnancy and lactation. During pregnancy, hormones from the placenta, including human placental lactogen (hPL), progesterone and oestrogens, act on the breast and stimulate proliferation of the alveolar tissue in preparation for lactation. The oestrogens prevent lactation from occurring during pregnancy. After parturition, when the influence of the placenta is removed, suckling of the baby stimulates the release of prolactin from the anterior pituitary, thereby stimulating milk formation, and release of oxytocin from the posterior pituitary, causing contraction of the smooth muscle around the alveoli and expelling milk from the breast.

the posterior pituitary. While prolactin stimulates milk formation, oxytocin stimulates the milk 'let down' reflex by causing contraction of the smooth muscle around the alveoli (milk ducts).

Self-assessment case study

Abnormal periods

A 14-year-old girl presented to her doctor with a lack of periods. Her menarche was at age 13 years, but she had had only two light periods before they stopped. She had not had a period for 8 months. She was generally well and was taking no medications. She lived with her parents and younger brother. Her school academic and sports performances were excellent, and she ran 10 km twice a week and cycled to and from school. There was no family history of note.

On examination, she looked well with a height of 1.74 m and a weight of 46 kg (body mass index 15.2 kg/m^2). Her skin, mouth, eyes, head and neck were normal. The pulse was 50 bpm and the blood pressure 110/65 mmHg.

The blood tests showed:

LH	1 U/L (normal 1–10 U/L)
FSH	1.2 U/L (normal 1–10 U/L)
Oestradiol	<75 pmol/L (normal 200–1200 pmol/L)
Testosterone	<1.2 nmol/L (normal 1.2–3.0 nmol/L)
Pregnancy test	Negative

Questions:

① How do you interpret the blood test?

② What other investigations may be helpful?

③ What is the differential diagnosis, starting with the likeliest?

Answers see page 148

Extended matching questions

A   Anorexia nervosa
B   Lactation
C   Menstrual cycle day 7
D   Menstrual cycle day 14
E   Menstrual cycle day 21
F   Menstrual cycle day 28
G   Polycystic ovarian syndrome (PCOS)
H   Pregnancy first trimester
I   Pregnancy second trimester
J   Pregnancy third trimester
K   Pre-menarche (absent puberty)
L   Post-menopause

For each of the following endocrine profiles from a 40-year-old woman who has previously had two normal pregnancies, select the most likely explanation from the list above:

① High oestradiol, low progesterone, high LH, high FSH levels.

② Very high progesterone, moderately high hCG, high hPL, very high prolactin levels.

③ Moderately high oestradiol, high progesterone, low LH, low FSH, undetectable hCG levels.

④ Normal oestradiol, very low progesterone, high LH/FSH ratio, high androstenedione, low SHBG levels.

⑤ High progesterone, high hCG, low hPL levels.

⑥ Low oestradiol, low progesterone, very high LH, very high FSH, undetectable hCG levels.

Answers see page 152

HORMONAL CONTROL OF REPRODUCTION PART III: SEX HORMONES DURING DEVELOPMENT

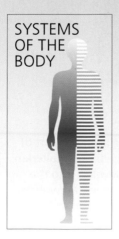

SYSTEMS OF THE BODY

Chapter objectives

After reading this chapter you should be able to:

① Explain the role of hormones in the control of sexual differentiation.

② Explain the concept of puberty and menarche.

③ Describe menopause and understand the use of hormone replacement therapy.

④ Understand how fertility may be regulated pharmacologically.

Introduction

Reproductive hormones are important for both sexes throughout life, starting with early fetal development where hormones have a key role in sexual differentiation. For teenagers, hormonal changes give rise to puberty. The previous chapters dealt with the role of hormones in reproduction. This chapter covers the role of hormones in early life and up to puberty, then, in later life, the hormonal changes of menopause and the use of hormone replacement therapy. It also considers how hormonal treatments can be used to modify fertility, both as contraceptive agents and as therapies designed to increase fertility.

Gender determination and differentiation

There are normally 46 chromosomes in human cells: 22 pairs of chromosomes plus two sex chromosomes, either XX or XY. The presence of two X chromosomes in a fetus leads to the development of ovaries, whereas the presence of one X and one Y chromosome leads to the development of testes. There is a gene on the short arm of the Y chromosome, termed sex determining region Y (*SRY*), but referred to as the 'testis determining factor', that causes a testis to develop. The product of the *SRY* gene is a DNA binding protein that is able to modify gene transcription directly, initiating a cascade of gene activation which is required for the development of a functional testis.

Until 6–7 weeks of gestation, however, there is no visible difference between a male and a female embryo. At this stage of embryonic development there is a primitive gonad which is found adjacent to two ducts, the mullerian ducts and the wolffian ducts (Fig. 8.1). These ducts will go on to form either the female reproductive tract (mullerian ducts) or the male reproductive tract (wolffian ducts). So at this stage the fetus has the potential to develop both sets of genitalia. It is the fetal gonad that determines whether the fetus develops the male or female phenotype (appearance). The default option is female genital development, and this is what is seen if the fetus either has ovaries or does not have a functional gonad. This is because no hormone secretion by the female gonad is needed for development of female genitalia: the mullerian ducts persist and differentiate to form the fallopian tubes, the uterus and the upper part of the vagina. The wolffian ducts simply regress.

Hormonal control of sexual differentiation

However, in order for male genitalia to develop there must be an active over-ride of the default option. It is testosterone that functions as this over-ride mechanism, in conjunction with a hormone called anti-mullerian hormone (AMH). Anti-mullerian hormone is a peptide hormone closely related to inhibin and activin. It is secreted by the Sertoli cells in the testis of the male fetus and its secretion continues after birth until about the age of 10 years.

Testosterone is secreted by the fetal Leydig cells and is converted to 5α-dihydrotestosterone (DHT). The DHT acts to stabilize the wolffian ducts, which can then develop into the epididymis, vas deferens and seminal vesicles of the male. DHT also acts to stimulate development of the male external genitalia. Meanwhile, the actions of AMH bring about regression of the mullerian ducts.

These events all take place over a relatively short period of time quite early in gestation so that sexual differentiation of the fetus is essentially complete by 12 weeks' gestation.

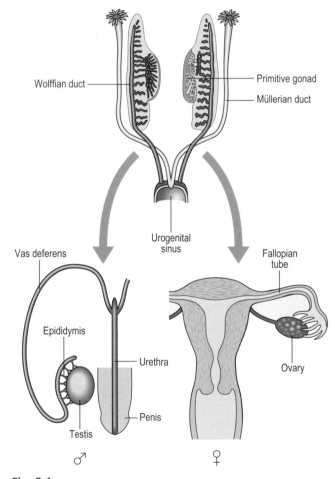

Fig. 8.1
The fetal primitive gonad showing the arrangement of wolffian and mullerian ducts. In the male, the mullerian ducts regress and the wolffian ducts develop into the epididymis and vas deferens. In the female, the wolffian ducts regress and the mullerian ducts develop to form the fallopian tubes.

Abonormalities of sexual differentiation

Abnormalities of sexual differentiation involving incorrect numbers of sex chromosomes are perhaps more common than you might think. Turner's syndrome is a condition in which a girl is born with only one X chromosome (denoted as 45XO), instead of the usual two. Although there is only one X chromosome, the fetus develops a female appearance with female genitalia because this is the 'default option' in the absence of a Y chromosome. It affects about 1 in 2000 newborn girls, although the great majority of fetuses with this abnormality do not survive past about week 28 of pregnancy. This is a serious condition which includes major abnormalities of the cardiovascular system as well as impaired ovarian function (Fig. 8.2). Women with Turner's syndrome do not usually go through normal pubertal development and menarche without medical intervention.

Klinefelter's syndrome affects about 1 in 800 newborn boys. These boys are born with an additional X chromosome (denoted as 47XXY), although there are cases where there are multiple additional copies of the X chromosome. Although they are phenotypically male and appear normal as infants, there is impaired testicular function. As adults, however, males with Klinefelter's syndrome are infertile. They have small testes, which are often undescended, and there is a varying degree of androgen deficiency, which is normally treated with testosterone replacement therapy. Thus it appears that the presence of a Y chromosome is sufficient to over-ride the default option during fetal development, but in the presence of more than one X chromosome it is not sufficient for normal testicular function.

There are other conditions that can give rise to a range of abnormalities, from ambiguous genitalia to true hermaphroditism. If a female fetus is exposed to high levels of testosterone, particularly before week 12 of fetal development, this can result in the development of 'ambiguous genitalia', as seen in congenital adrenal hyperplasia (see Chapter 4). The androgens cause masculinization of the genitals, resulting in an enlarged clitoris and fusion of the labial folds.

Defects of the *SRY* gene have been reported in patients with a normal 46XY karyotype. This usually results in the formation of female external genitalia, but can present as a male phenotype with underdeveloped external genitalia. In both cases there is significant abnormality of the gonads, with infertility and a greatly increased risk of gonadal tumour development. The treatment is therefore to remove the gonads and to give sex steroids appropriate to the phenotype at puberty.

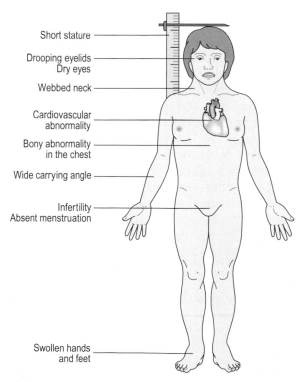

Short stature

Drooping eyelids
Dry eyes

Webbed neck

Cardiovascular
abnormality

Bony abnormality
in the chest

Wide carrying angle

Infertility
Absent menstruation

Swollen hands
and feet

Fig. 8.2
Features of Turner's syndrome (karyotype 45XO). In addition to the features shown, there is failure of normal pubertal development. The swelling of the hands and feet is due to lymphatic abnormalities.

Interesting fact

There has been concern over recent years about chemicals in the environment. Many industrial processes create chemicals with either oestrogen-like or anti-androgenic properties. There is, in addition, a considerable amount of oestrogen that ends up in river water downstream of sewage treatment plants. This comes from the urine of both normally cycling women and women taking the oral contraceptive pill. The effect of these chemicals in the environment has been to cause abnormal sexual differentiation in both fish and higher mammals. Male fish, living downstream of sewage treatment plants, have been found to develop an intersex gonad, containing both spermatogonia and eggs, although the eggs are not fertile. In the Arctic, there have also been reports of polar bears (who are at the top of the food chain and therefore likely to get a higher 'dose' of such chemicals) with both male and female sex organs: the true hermaphrodite state. The media has tagged the chemicals causing these effects 'gender benders'.

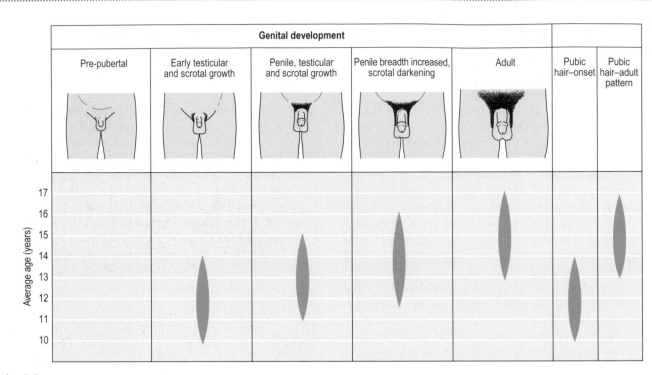

Fig. 8.3
Stages of pubertal genital and pubic hair development in boys, with the average age of each stage shown.

We do not know whether these agents also affect people. It is clear that there is an increased incidence of relatively minor developmental abnormalities in boys. These include cryptorchidism, where one or both testes have not descended into the scrotum, and hypospadias, where the urethral opening is halfway down the penis, instead of at the tip where it is usually found. There is also a well documented decrease in sperm quality in men living in developed countries over the past 50 years. However, it is not at all clear whether these effects can be explained by increased exposure to environmental chemicals, particularly given the huge changes in lifestyle and other environmental factors over this time period.

Hormones during development: puberty and menarche

It is not clear exactly what the hormonal signal is that triggers the start of puberty. There are various theories, but it is still not certain what removes the 'brake' on gonadotropin releasing hormone (GnRH) secretion by the hypothalamus. What is known is that the hypothalamus in pre-pubertal children is exceptionally sensitive to the negative feedback effect of the sex steroids, and the low steroid levels found in children are sufficient to inhibit the axis. There also

appears to be a requirement for the maturation of GnRH secretory mechanisms before puberty can occur.

As mentioned in previous chapters, the pituitary hormones luteinizing hormone (LH) and follicle stimulating hormone (FSH) are effectively stimulated only by pulses of GnRH. Although GnRH is secreted in a pulsatile manner throughout childhood, there is an increase in both the amplitude and the frequency of these pulses at puberty. It has been suggested that the pulse-generator in the brain is the key regulator of puberty. The net effect is that, with the removal of the hypersensitivity to feedback inhibition and the increased amplitude and frequency of GnRH pulses, LH and FSH secretion is increased, leading to greatly increased secretion of sex steroids by the gonads. This increase in oestrogen in girls and in testosterone in boys brings about the physical changes associated with puberty.

Pubertal development in boys

In boys, the first sign of puberty is an increase in the size of the testes which occurs as a result of increased FSH secretion, usually around the age of 10–12 years (Fig. 8.3). This is followed by an increase in size of the penis and a change in the colour and size of the scrotum, which continues until adult proportions are attained by the age of about 16 years. Pubic hair begins to appear during genital development after the enlargement of the testes. The growth spurt associated

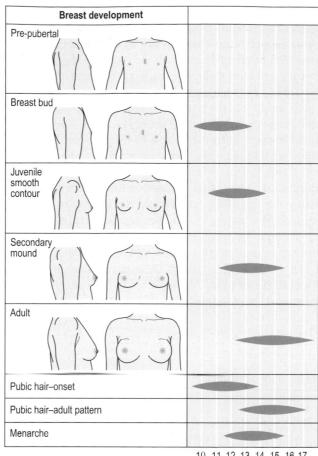

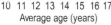

Fig. 8.4
Stages of pubertal development in girls, with the average age of each stage shown.

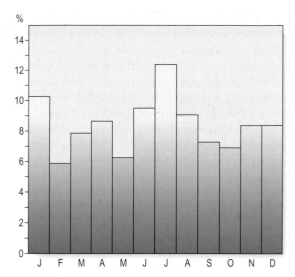

Fig. 8.5
These data from the USA show that there is seasonal variation in the frequency of menarche. The graph shows the percentage of the study group of nearly 3000 girls recording menarche in each month. There were almost twice as many instances of menarche in July compared with February. The average should be about 8.3% if menarche is evenly distributed through the year. There was no relation found between birth month and month of menarche. (Data taken from Matchock R L, Susman E J, Brown F M 2004 Women's Health Issues **14**: 184–192.)

with puberty usually starts about 12 months after the first sign of puberty is noted and continues through the second half of pubertal development. The development of the genitalia occurs in parallel with development of pubic and axillary hair, and both are under the control of androgens.

Pubertal development in girls

In girls, the onset of puberty is heralded by the beginning of breast development, which usually occurs from about the age of 10 years (Fig. 8.4). Pubic hair begins to develop at about the same time. Pubic hair development is usually complete by about the age of 15–16 years and breast development by the age of 16–17 years. The age of menarche (the first menstrual period) is determined by many factors including genetics, body weight, family size and season of the year (Fig. 8.5). Over the past century there has been a progressive decline in the average age of menarche in the developed world. This has been suggested to result from a decreased incidence of childhood illness together with improved nutrition of children. The average age of menarche is currently about 13 years (with a normal range of 11–15 years), although there is some geographical variation.

Interesting fact

The decrease in the average age of menarche in the developed world since the mid-19th century, from 14–15 to 12–13 years, has been well documented. This has been attributed to improvements in diet and general health. However, what is not generally reported is that records from ancient Greece show that the average age of menarche at this time was 12–14 years. Similarly, in classical Indian civilizations (500 BC to AD 500) the average age of menarche was 12–13 years, compared with 13–14 years in modern India. The implication is that early industrialization and urbanization is associated with a shift to a later menarche, whereas later stages of economic development bring the age of menarche back down to pre-industrial levels.

Disorders of puberty

The onset of puberty can be delayed by several factors, including low body weight and excessive exercise, both of which are often features of anorexia nervosa. When anorexia nervosa is found in adult women there is often a return to pre-pubertal patterns of gonadotropin secretion. Amenorrhoea (failure of menstruation) is common in these disorders, as we have already seen in Chapter 7. There are additionally several much less common endocrine causes of delayed puberty such as androgen insensitivity syndrome and hypogonadotropic hypogonadism (see, for example, the case of John Smith in Chapter 6).

Delayed puberty is clinically significant. The epiphyses of the long bones fuse only under the influence of sex steroids produced during puberty, so a delay in puberty can result in excessive long bone growth. On the other hand, sex steroids are essential for effective mineralization of bones at puberty, and the absence of puberty can result in significant bone weakness. There are some very unpleasant cases of bone fractures being seen in female gymnasts whose exercise regimes have had the effect of delaying puberty, thus causing weakness of bone structure.

It is less usual for early or 'precocious' puberty to be seen. In boys, precocious puberty is defined as pubertal development before the age of 9 years and requires investigation. In girls, early puberty is fairly common and tends to run in families. It is not usually due to an identifiable abnormality and, unless puberty occurs before the age of 6 years, would not normally be investigated. One cause of precocious puberty is congenital adrenal hyperplasia, in which excessive adrenal androgen secretion causes abnormal early genital development. This might be a good time to re-read the case history in Chapter 4 with the benefit of your increased knowledge of the reproductive system.

Amenorrhoea box 1

Case history

Maria Lobo, a 32-year-old woman, attended for her annual review in an endocrine outpatient clinic 2 years after the successful treatment of her Graves' disease. She was worried that she may have a recurrence of her overactive thyroid gland because she had been experiencing increasingly frequent flushing and palpitations since before her last checkup. However, she also mentioned that her periods, which had become irregular 18 months ago, had stopped completely about 10 months ago. She had even bought a home pregnancy test, but this was negative.

Mrs Lobo had entered puberty and had her first menstrual period at the age of about 13 years. She had had two normal pregnancies with vaginal deliveries at the age of 23 and 26 years. She was taking no medication and used barrier methods of contraception. She exercised for about 60 minutes a week and ate a normal balanced diet. The family history was positive for autoimmune disease, with her mother and sister also having Graves' disease.

On examination, she was somewhat thin, with a weight of 56.3 kg and a body mass index of 20.6 kg/m^2. The thyroid was not enlarged. She was clinically euthyroid with a pulse of 75 beats per minute. Secondary sexual characteristics including breast and pubic hair development were normal. The remainder of the examination was normal.

What investigations should you request and why?

Menopause and the climacteric

Just as menarche marks the start of a woman's reproductive life, so menopause marks the end. After the menopause (the term applied to a woman's final menstrual period), normal pregnancy is not possible. Menopause is generally defined as the permanent cessation of menstruation as a result of the loss of ovarian follicles. It requires 12 months of amenorrhoea and can therefore be identified only with hindsight. Just as menarche is a single event within puberty, so menopause is a single event within the 'climacteric'. This is the term applied to the period of transition between pre-menopausal and post-menopausal states. In lay terms the climacteric is often referred to as 'the change'.

Until the 20th century, little was known about the menopause and the health of post-menopausal women, partly because relatively few women lived beyond their reproductive lifespan. It has also been suggested that the almost exclusively male doctors of the 19th century were more influenced by prevailing cultural stereotypes than by scientific evidence. Because menopause was seen as the end of a woman's 'useful' life, the menopause was associated with diagnoses such as 'feeble mindedness' and 'involutional melancholia' for which there was no evidence base.

It is perhaps surprising that, despite significant changes in life expectancy and a marked decrease in the age of menarche over the past century, there does not appear to have been any change at all in the average age at which women reach the menopause. The median age of menopause is 51 years and average life expectancy for women in the UK is currently about 80 years, giving a woman around 30 years of post-menopausal life.

Menopause occurs naturally as a result of the ovaries running out of follicles. The ovarian follicles degenerate and disappear, a process called atresia. It can therefore be seen as a physiological form of ovarian failure. This is usually not a condition of sudden onset. The ovaries become less sensitive to LH and FSH stimulation over a period of a few years with a gradual decline in oestrogen production. Premature ovarian failure can be medically induced as a consequence of either chemotherapy or radiotherapy. It may also be surgically induced by bilateral oophorectomy (removal of both ovaries).

Interesting fact

It is only women who experience the end of their reproductive lives so long before the end of their lifespan. It is thought that this reflects the fact that women are born with their total number of follicles, which cannot be increased. Men, on the other hand, have relatively unlimited capacity for spermatogenesis and usually continue to produce sperm throughout their lives, although there are concerns about the quality of sperm produced by older men. Females of other species remain reproductively active for a greater proportion of their lives. Various theories have been proposed to explain this, but it may be a reflection of the length of time it takes for a human to reach sexual maturity and independence, compared with the young of other species.

Premature ovarian failure

This is defined as spontaneous ovarian failure occurring before the age of 40 years; it affects around 1% of women. The reasons for premature menopause are not well understood but it seems likely that it may result from either a smaller than usual number of follicles formed during fetal development, or an increased rate of follicular loss after birth. It is not clear how either of these situations occurs. In both cases the number of follicles falls below a critical level at an earlier age than normal, resulting in primary ovarian failure.

There are other causes of primary ovarian failure, including autoimmune destruction of the ovaries.

Amenorrhoea box 2

Case note: Investigations

The following investigations were performed:

Pregnancy test	Result negative
Serum free T4	Normal
Serum TSH	Normal
Serum oestradiol	Low
Serum LH	Very high
Serum FSH	Very high
Autoantibody screen	Positive for thyroid peroxidase antibodies

All women of child-bearing age with amenorrhoea should first be assumed to be pregnant and a pregnancy test must be performed.

In view of her past history of Graves' disease, thyroid function should be checked even though Mrs Lobo is clinically euthyroid. Mrs Lobo has amenorrhoea, which could be due to primary ovarian failure or be secondary to reduced gonadotropin secretion. These can be distinguished by measuring oestradiol, LH and FSH levels. If the levels are all low, the cause is failure of gonadotropin secretion. However, Mrs Lobo's results show a low oestradiol concentration and very high levels of LH and FSH, indicating primary ovarian failure. Finally, the strong family history suggests that autoimmune diseases attacking the endocrine organs may be present in her and her family. Therefore, autoimmune disease of the ovary is a possible cause.

The presence of anti-thyroid peroxidase autoantibodies would fit with the idea that the ovarian failure is due to an autoimmune attack. Unfortunately, anti-ovarian auto-antibodies cannot be measured reliably, and so cannot be used to confirm the diagnosis.

What is the diagnosis?

Symptoms of the menopause

The acute symptoms of the menopause are usually attributed to the marked decline in circulating oestrogen seen during menopause. These symptoms can be divided into three groups: vasomotor, sexual and psychological (Box 8.1). It is not clear whether the psychological symptoms, other than decreased libido, are the result of decreased circulating oestrogen, or whether they may reflect other life changes occurring at that time, such as children gaining independence, for example.

> **Box 8.1**
>
> ## Acute symptoms of the menopause
>
> **Vasomotor**
>
> Hot flushes
> Night sweats
>
> **Sexual**
>
> Vaginal dryness leading to painful intercourse
> Increased incidence of urinary tract and vaginal
> infections
>
> **Psychological**
>
> Decreased libido (sex drive)
> Anxiety, labile mood

The major early symptoms of the menopause are hot flushes and night sweats. These are due to vasodilatation in the skin with a rise in skin temperature and sweating. The flushes are often felt in the upper body, head and neck, but also occur all over the body, and may be associated with palpitations. They may occur multiple times a day. Flushing occurs in any cause of hypogonadism where there has previously been some sex hormone exposure.

There are significant cultural differences in women's experience of the menopause. In Britain and the USA approximately 70% of women report night sweating and hot flushes (called hot flashes in the USA). In other cultures, this percentage is lower. It has been suggested that diet and lifestyle may be important in determining the severity of menopausal symptoms. The oriental diet, for example, is rich in soy, which contains plant oestrogens, believed by some to minimize the effects of the menopause.

There are, in addition, significant long-term consequences of the menopause. Osteoporosis is a major problem in post-menopausal women. Oestrogen deficiency results in a significant year-on-year decrease in bone mass, at a rate of about 1–2% of total bone mass each year. Although men also lose bone as they get older, it happens much faster in women, with the effect that about 1 in 3 older women has osteoporosis, compared with 1 in 12 men. Osteoporosis results in a significantly increased risk of fracture (see Chapter 10).

The effects of oestrogen deficiency on the urinary and genital tracts can result in vaginal prolapse and urinary incontinence. This, together with vaginal dryness, leads to an increased frequency of urinary tract infections.

It is generally considered that oestrogens are protective against heart disease. This is reflected in the significantly lower incidence of myocardial infarction in women compared to men. The incidence of heart disease in women increases significantly after the menopause, although the reason for this is unclear. Our current understanding is that hormone replacement therapy does not significantly alter the incidence of heart disease in post-menopausal women, suggesting that it is not simply a direct effect of oestrogens.

> **Amenorrhoea box 3**
>
> ### Case note: Diagnosis
>
> Mrs Lobo had ovarian failure at the age of 32 years, and therefore had premature ovarian failure, which is defined as ovarian failure occurring spontaneously below the age of 40 years. The symptoms are the same as normal menopause. Iatrogenic premature ovarian failure may be a consequence of surgery, chemotherapy or radiotherapy. The causes of premature ovarian failure differ depending on the age of the patient. Genetic or chromosomal abnormalities usually result in failure of the ovary to develop and present with a lack of puberty and primary amenorrhoea (i.e. the patient has never had a menstrual period).
>
> In Mrs Lobo, the ovaries had developed normally, she had had two successful pregnancies and there was a later destruction of the ovaries by the auto-immune disease process. Primary ovarian failure is part of the spectrum of organ-specific autoimmune diseases. In order to confirm the diagnosis, an ovarian biopsy could have been performed via a laparoscope inserted into the peritoneum and pelvis. However, this was considered invasive and Mrs Lobo preferred not to have this done.
>
> By definition, Mrs Lobo was in the climacteric, with premature ovarian failure, perimenopausal symptoms and no periods for 10 months. By the time the investigations were completed and she attended her next appointment, she had not had a period for a year, so the end of her last period was retrospectively designated the start of her menopause.

Table 8.1
Comparison of typical formulations of the oral contraceptive pill, HRT and the morning-after pill

Preparation	Oestrogen	Progestin
Oral contraceptive	Ethinyloestradiol 35 μg	Norethisterone 500 μg or levonorgestrel 150 μg
HRT	Conjugated equine oestradiol 1 mg	Norethisterone 1 mg
Morning-after pill	None	Levonorgestrel 2 × 750 μg

Structures of the synthetic steroids are shown in Figure 8.6. Although a larger amount of oestrogen is used in HRT compared with that in the oral contraceptive pill, the conjugated oestrogen is much less potent than ethinyloestradiol.

Hormone replacement therapy

It is clear that the menopause causes significant health problems in both the short and the long term. The use of hormone replacement therapy (HRT) to treat these problems is a controversial issue.

HRT is the term given to the use of oestrogens to treat menopausal symptoms. In a woman with an intact uterus, oestrogen administration causes an increased risk of uterine cancer. This risk can be reversed by the inclusion of progesterone in the HRT. So, for a woman with a uterus, 'combination HRT' is used, but oestrogen alone can be given following hysterectomy. A comparison of the dosage regimens typically used for HRT and the oral contraceptive pill is shown in Table 8.1 and the structures of the steroids used are shown in Figure 8.6.

HRT is very good at treating the early effects of the menopause, preventing both hot flushes and night sweats. Many women find that this also has a significant effect on their psychological symptoms, but it is not clear whether this is a direct effect or a secondary benefit from an improved quality of life resulting from better sleep. It is also clear that HRT improves sexual function, improving both vaginal lubrication and libido.

Long-term HRT

More controversial are the effects of HRT on the long-term consequences of the menopause. As with the drug treatment of any condition, there is a risk:benefit ratio to be considered. In the case of HRT the risks are still unclear. It has been hotly debated as to whether HRT causes an increased or decreased risk of cardiovascular disease. There have been large studies that have reported only marginal effects, so it seems likely that any risk, or indeed any benefit, is minimal.

One of the main reasons for long-term use of HRT is the prevention of osteoporosis. The rate of bone loss can be reduced significantly by taking HRT, and this is reflected in the lower rate of bone fracture in long-term HRT users. However, this protective effect lasts

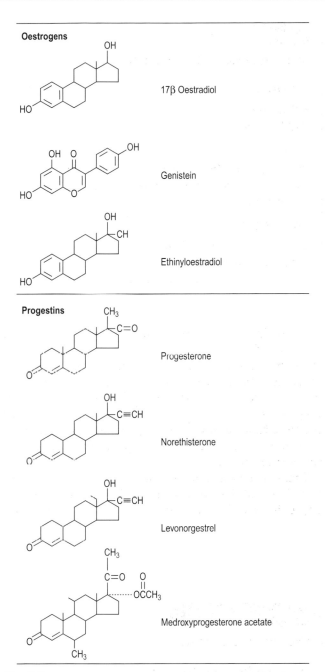

Fig. 8.6
Structures of steroids commonly used in contraception and HRT, together with genistein, a plant oestrogen. The only difference between 17β-oestradiol and ethinyloestradiol is the ethinyl group added at C17. However, this small structural change makes an enormous difference to the activity of the steroid; ethinyloestradiol does not bind significantly to sex hormone binding globulin (SHBG), unlike oestradiol, and undergoes very little first-pass metabolism in the liver. It is the most potent oestrogen currently available. Both norethisterone and levonorgestrel have the properties of a progestin, but structurally resemble a cross between progesterone and ethinyloestradiol.

only as long as the HRT is taken. Once it is stopped, bone loss resumes at the same rate it would in the absence of HRT. It has been suggested that HRT may also prevent the development of neurodegenerative diseases such as Alzheimer's disease. However, despite several studies there is no reliable evidence to support this suggestion.

It is clear that taking HRT causes an increased risk of breast cancer and that this risk goes up further the longer that HRT is used. It is for this reason that many women choose to take HRT for 1 or 2 years, to treat the early menopausal symptoms, and then move to alternative therapies to prevent osteoporosis.

Alternative therapies

There is a variety of alternatives to taking HRT for the long-term treatment of menopausal symptoms. Osteoporosis may be prevented by a diet rich in calcium

Box 8.2

Risks and benefits of long-term HRT use

Benefits

- Sexual health – HRT maintains vaginal structure and lubrication, and increases libido
- Bone health – HRT maintains bone mineral density and so reduces risk of osteoporosis
- HRT has also been suggested to improve cognitive function, wound healing and eye health
- HRT may also reduce the risk of cardiovascular disease, Alzheimer's disease and colonic cancer

Risks

- Breast cancer – HRT is associated with an increased risk of breast cancer
- Deep vein thrombosis – HRT causes a small increase in the risk of DVT
- Endometrial cancer – This risk is associated with oestrogen-only forms of HRT

Amenorrhoea box 4

Case note: Future health risks

The main consequence of failure of ovarian hormone production is oestrogen deficiency, although the levels of other steroids, including some male sex steroids, also decline. The main effects of oestrogen deficiency are clinical symptoms and effects on bone mineralization. The lack of oestrogen results in loss of bone mineral, leading to osteoporosis and a risk of osteoporotic fractures. Dual-energy X-ray absorptiometry (DEXA) of bone mineral density is a useful guide to deciding whether osteoporosis is present.

The aims of treatment are to alleviate symptoms and prevent post-menopausal fractures. The main treatment used for Mrs Lobo was hormone replacement therapy with a combined oestrogen and progestogen preparation. Unfortunately, full HRT is associated with increased risks in patients above the age of 50 years (Box 8.2). The risk of endometrial cancer can be reduced by opposing oestrogens with progestogens. Bile cholesterol is increased in oestrogen-treated women and this worsens gallbladder disease. Some patients may still prefer full HRT if they have severe symptoms or advancing osteoporosis after the age of 50 years. A daily supplement of oral calcium should be added to Mrs Lobo's regimen. The bisphosphonates are effective at reducing osteoclast action, improving bone density and reducing fractures. They should be used if there is osteoporosis.

HRT also has benefits for libido and vaginal secretion.

and vitamin D, regular exercise and the use of bisphosphonates. These regimens have been shown to have as much effect as HRT in preventing post-menopausal bone loss and appear to have fewer side effects.

Sexual dysfunction, such as vaginal dryness and discomfort, can be readily relieved by the use of a simple water-based lubricant jelly.

Some foods, including soy products, contain high levels of plant oestrogens (phyto-oestrogens) and various preparations of these are sold in health food shops. These are often marketed as 'alternative therapies' for menopausal symptoms, although there is no conclusive evidence that they work.

Interesting fact

According to the Bible, Abraham's wife, Sarah, was 90 years old when she became pregnant. This was, at the time, considered miraculous, but current records for the oldest woman to conceive are being broken every year as a result of advances in in-vitro fertilization (IVF) techniques. Proponents argue that it is a woman's right to conceive after normal menopause and point out that in previous centuries, when life expectancy was lower, it was usual for women to die before menopause. Opponents argue that there are good physical and psychological reasons why menopause occurs when it does and that pregnancy after this age is unnatural. What do you think?

Hormonal control of fertility: contraception

Oral contraceptive agents have a long history. In ancient Greece both pomegranate seeds and penny-royal plants were used as oral contraceptives. In the seventh century BC a plant called silphium was in great demand as a result of its reputation as a highly effective contraceptive. It was exported from its native North Africa in such large quantities that by the fourth century AD it was extinct. We will never know what the active component of silphium might have been, but all the orally active contraceptive agents in use today are based on derivatives of steroid hormones.

During the middle part of the 20th century the great increase in our knowledge and understanding of the role of hormones in reproduction led directly to the development of hormonal methods of contraception. These fairly rapidly became the most popular method of contraception in the developed world. Until now, all hormonal methods of contraception have been designed for use by women. A 'male pill' has been undergoing development for at least three decades, but none is currently available.

The oral contraceptive pill

This is usually a combination of an oestrogen and a progestogen, although sometimes a 'progestogen only' pill is used. The steroids are usually synthetic versions of the naturally occurring hormones; the synthetic oestrogen is usually ethinyloestradiol and there are various synthetic progestogens in use, including norethindrone (norethisterone) and levonorgestrel (see Fig. 8.6). There are various combinations available and different schedules of administration, with perhaps the most common being the '21 days on, 7 days off' method.

The oral contraceptive pill works by mimicking the natural gonadal steroids and exerting feedback inhibition on the hypothalamo–pituitary–gonadal axis. This inhibits hypothalamic GnRH release and blocks pituitary LH and FSH release. In the absence of LH and FSH, there is no follicular development and so ovulation does not occur. The oral pill is also thought to cause thickening of the cervical mucus, presenting a physical barrier to sperm reaching the uterus.

The contraceptive pill is taken once daily. Its efficacy relies on efficient entero-hepatic recycling of steroids: steroids are conjugated in the liver and secreted in bile into the gastrointestinal tract, where they are de-conjugated and reabsorbed into the blood. This cycle is disrupted by certain antibiotics and by gastrointestinal disturbance, making the oral contraceptive pill much less effective at these times. Otherwise it is

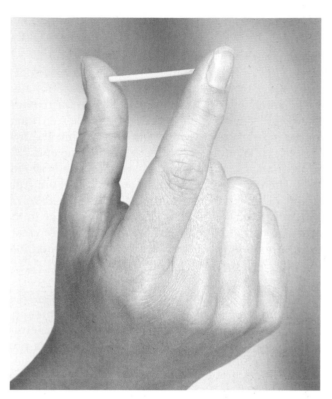

Fig. 8.7
Contraceptive implant. (Courtesy of Organon.)

an extremely effective and reliable form of contraception, and is well tolerated by most women.

Long-term contraception

As an alternative to taking a daily 'pill', there are several long-acting hormonal contraceptive preparations available. There are two main forms of long-term contraception: the oily preparation of a progestogen, which is slowly hydrolysed, and the implant, which slowly releases progestogens (Fig. 8.7). These work on the same basis as the oral contraceptive pill but are administered much less frequently. The injectable forms last 3 months on average, whereas the implant lasts for up to a year. This form of contraceptive is not yet widely used, but the most common form of injectable contraceptive is Depo-Provera (medroxyprogesterone acetate). The efficacy of these preparations is not affected by stomach upsets or by other medication, and because there is no question of 'forgetting to take a pill' their efficacy is very nearly 100%. There are some side effects, particularly 'breakthrough bleeding', although a new generation of combination implants has been developed to overcome this problem.

There are, in addition, a number of intra-uterine contraceptive devices available whose efficacy has been improved by the inclusion of a hormonal implant.

Emergency hormonal contraception

The morning-after pill

A high dose of combined oestrogen and progestogen is used to prevent a pregnancy in the 72 hours after sexual intercourse has taken place. The effectiveness of this pill depends on how long after sexual intercourse it is taken. It is most effective within the first 24 hours. If taken up to 72 hours later, it prevents 75% of pregnancies, but it is much less effective after this time. The mechanism of action of this pill is not fully understood, but there is thought to be an alkalinization of the fluid within the uterus and a change in the structure of the endometrium, which together create an environment that is unfavourable for implantation.

Anti-progestogens

As pregnancy is dependent on fairly constant levels of circulating progesterone, one method of terminating an early pregnancy is the use of the anti-progesterone called RU486, or mifepristone. Mifepristone is a progesterone receptor antagonist, which prevents progesterone from binding to its receptor. It is effective both as a morning-after pill and for inducing termination of pregnancy at a later stage. It is an effective alternative to the surgical termination of pregnancy, which is the most commonly used method. The fact that mifepristone is not widely used is due more to political than to clinical considerations.

A male contraceptive pill?

There has been considerable progress towards developing a hormonal contraceptive for use by men. The approach has been to try to develop a regimen of hormone delivery that will inhibit hypothalamic GnRH release, as in the female contraceptive pill. Testosterone itself is the ideal candidate for this purpose, as it would allow potency and secondary sexual characteristics to be maintained. Supra-physiological doses of testosterone have an inhibitory effect on the hypothalamus and pituitary, shutting off androgen production in the testis and preventing sperm production. The main problem is that testosterone and other androgens cause liver damage when taken by mouth. To try to get round this, a testosterone skin patch has been developed. Most patches also contain

a progestogen, as the combination of steroids is much more effective than testosterone alone. Several trials of these patches have been conducted but they are not yet available commercially.

Hormonal control of fertility: assisted conception

A woman who is not able to conceive naturally may undergo a number of investigations, including measurements of LH, FSH, prolactin, progesterone and testosterone. A woman who is not ovulating normally may be treated with a drug designed to stimulate ovulation.

Simple induction of ovulation

Clomifene is an anti-oestrogen. It binds to oestrogen receptors and blocks the action of oestrogens in the circulation. It has been known since the early 1960s that clomifene stimulates the release of gonadotropins and so can stimulate ovulation. Usually this treatment results in the production of only one or two eggs at a time, but occasionally can result in multiple births.

Preparation for IVF treatment or egg donation

Hormonal treatments can be used to make a woman produce multiple eggs in a single cycle. These eggs are then harvested and used for IVF. The treatment has three phases. The first drug used is buserelin, a GnRH agonist, which is delivered as a nasal spray. By providing the pituitary with a constant stimulation, instead of the usual pulsatile GnRH, gonadotropin secretion is turned off. After 2 weeks of this treatment, when the hypothalamo–pituitary–gonadal axis is thoroughly shut down, FSH is given by daily injection for about 10 days to stimulate egg development. At the end of the 10-day treatment, ovulation is induced with a single injection of chorionic gonadotropin (hCG) and the eggs are 'harvested' 36 hours later. Typically this treatment produces 6 to 12 eggs.

The harvested eggs are mixed with sperm and then implanted in the uterus about 36 hours after fertilization.

Self-assessment case study

A case of lack of puberty and short stature

A 17-year-old girl presented with a lack of periods. She had been short since childhood, always being the smallest in her class. She had not developed breasts or pubic hair and had never had a period.

On examination, her height was 147 cm. There was an increased carrying angle at the elbow and she had no secondary sexual characteristics. There was a systolic ejection murmur over the left upper chest and the blood pressure was 175/115 mmHg.

The investigations showed:

Pregnancy test	Negative
Oestradiol	<75 pmol/L (normal 200–1200 pmol/L)
LH	>75 U/L (normal 1–10 U/L)
FSH	>75 U/L (normal 1–10 U/L)
Prolactin	360 mU/L (normal <400 mU/L)
Growth hormone	<0.5 mU/L (normal <0.5 mU/L in daytime)
Insulin-like growth factor 1	35 ng/mL (normal range for her age 130–330 ng/mL)

Questions:

① What is the diagnosis?

② What is the cause of the cardiac murmur and raised blood pressure?

③ What test confirms the diagnosis?

④ Will she have periods when treated with hormone replacement therapy?

⑤ Will she be fertile?

Answers see page 148

Extended matching questions

A   Bisphosphonates
B   Buserelin
C   Clomifene
D   Conjugated equine oestradiol
E   Ethinyloestradiol
F   Genistein
G   KY jelly
H   Medroxyprogesterone acetate
I   Methyltestosterone
J   Mifepristone (RU486)
K   Norethisterone
L   Silphium

For each of the definitions below, choose the substance that best fits from the list above:

① This synthetic progestin is used as an injectable female contraceptive.

② This progesterone receptor antagonist can be used as a morning-after pill.

③ This anti-oestrogen is used to stimulate ovulation in fertility treatment.

④ This GnRH agonist can be given as a nasal spray in fertility treatment.

⑤ This phyto-oestrogen is marketed as a 'complementary' form of HRT.

⑥ This progestin is commonly used in the oral contraceptive pill.

Answers see page 152

INSULIN AND THE REGULATION OF PLASMA GLUCOSE

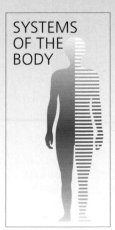

SYSTEMS OF THE BODY

Chapter objectives

After reading this chapter you should be able to:

① Explain how plasma glucose concentrations are maintained within a normal range.

② Explain the mechanisms controlling the secretion of insulin.

③ Describe the actions of insulin.

④ Explain the consequences of a deficiency in insulin production or action.

⑤ Describe the main treatment options for type 1 and type 2 diabetes mellitus.

⑥ Describe the 'metabolic syndrome'.

Introduction

The brain uses glucose, its main energy source, at a much faster rate than any other tissue in the body (Fig. 9.1). It is perhaps surprising, therefore, that the brain does not keep significant stores of glucose. Instead the brain relies on obtaining a constant supply of glucose from the blood. As a result, the brain is extremely sensitive to a fall in blood glucose levels. On the other hand, a sustained high level of blood glucose causes problems due to the increased osmolarity of blood; ultimately this leads to tissue damage as a result of inappropriate glycosylation in body tissues. Circulating concentrations of glucose are therefore maintained within relatively tight limits. This requires a complex system of control because plasma glucose levels can rise rapidly after a meal, but can also become very low during periods of fasting.

There are several hormones that act to increase circulating glucose concentrations, but the major hormone involved in lowering blood glucose load is insulin, a hormone secreted by the pancreas. A deficiency of either insulin production or effectiveness results in a condition known as *diabetes mellitus*. There are two forms of this disorder: type 1, which is insulin dependent (IDDM) and results from loss of insulin production; and type 2 or 'non-insulin-dependent' (NIDDM),

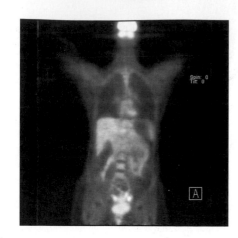

Fig. 9.1
Whole-body fluoro-deoxyglucose positron emission tomography (FDG-PET) scan, showing sites of glucose uptake, obtained following administration of a derivative of glucose as a 'tracer'. The main 'hotspot' of glucose uptake is clearly the brain. Although it looks as though the bladder is also a hotspot, this is only because the tracer is being excreted in the urine. (Courtesy Dr Norbert Avril, Department of Nuclear Medicine, St Bartholomew's Hospital.)

Table 9.1
Differences between insulin-dependent diabetes mellitus and non-insulin-dependent diabetes mellitus

	Type 1 (IDDM)	Type 2 (NIDDM)
Age at presentation (years)	<40	>40
Weight	Low/normal	Obese
Genetics	HLA linkage	Strong family history
Plasma insulin	Low	High
Ketoacidosis risk	High	Low

Interesting fact

The word 'insulin' comes from the Latin 'insula', meaning island, because insulin is produced by the islands of endocrine cells (islets of Langerhans) scattered throughout the pancreas.

Type 1 diabetes mellitus box 1

Case history

Robert Smith was an 18-year-old student. He had arrived at his first term of university feeling tired. He initially attributed this to an increased consumption of alcohol in the first 2 weeks, but he still felt tired when he stopped drinking. The next symptom was passing a lot of urine. He needed to pass urine frequently in the day and six times during the night. The urine volume was always large. He also noticed increased thirst and would go to bed with a 1.5-litre bottle of soft drink to quench his thirst. He was regularly buying soft drinks during the day. He finally went to see the university health centre doctor when he found his clothes were loose and realized he was losing weight. It was noted that his breath smelled ketotic, a characteristic sickly sweet smell that denotes an excess of ketones in the blood.

When Robert arrived at the university health centre, a nurse asked him to pass a sample of urine for testing and took his weight (60 kg), height (1.75 metres), pulse (90 beats per min) and blood pressure (115/75 mmHg). The following results were found:

Body mass index (BMI – height in metres/[weight in kg]^2) – 19.6 m/kg^2 (normal range 20–25 m/kg^2)

Urine dipstick testing: glucose +++, ketones ++

After learning Robert's story and getting the test results, the doctor immediately told him that the diagnosis was insulin-dependent diabetes mellitus.

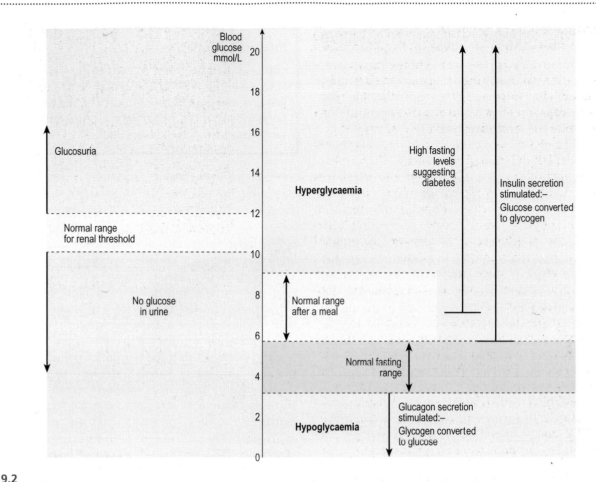

Fig. 9.2
This diagram shows the normal range of fasting blood glucose and the normal levels after a meal. A fasting blood glucose above 7 mmol/L suggests diabetes mellitus. Glucosuria is seen when the blood glucose level exceeds the renal threshold, which is usually around 10–12 mmol/L, but is very variable. When the blood glucose concentration increases above the normal fasting range of 3–5 mmol/L, insulin secretion is stimulated, and levels below this range cause glucagon secretion to increase. These two hormones act to maintain blood glucose levels within the normal range.

which is a condition of insulin resistance (Table 9.1). This chapter is concerned mainly with type 1 diabetes mellitus.

Glucose in urine

Blood glucose levels are normally maintained at around 3–5 mmol/L in the fasting state. After a meal this can rise to 7–8 mmol/L, but does not normally exceed about 10 mmol/L (Fig. 9.2). Above this level of blood glucose, the 'renal threshold' may be exceeded, with the result that glucose appears in the urine. Normally glucose, as a small molecule, passes through the kidney filtration mechanism into the urine and is then reabsorbed as the filtrate passes through the renal tubules. This mechanism involves active transport of glucose out of the urine and is facilitated by

a glucose transporter, which works well at normal blood glucose concentrations, so that all the glucose is reabsorbed and none appears in the urine. At high blood glucose concentrations the transporter mechanism becomes saturated, with the result that not all of the glucose can be reabsorbed and glucose appears in the urine. This is called glycosuria, which can be detected easily and rapidly with a Multistick test. The presence of glucose in urine may suggest a problem with glycaemic control, such as diabetes mellitus.

The term 'renal threshold' refers to the minimum level of blood glucose that results in glycosuria. It is worth noting that the renal threshold varies greatly both between individuals and as a result of different conditions. For example, in pregnancy there is often a fall in renal threshold and glycosuria may be seen, without necessarily indicating a problem. Conversely, renal threshold increases with age and diabetes mellitus may not result in glycosuria in older people.

When glucose does appear in the urine, this causes an osmotic diuresis, resulting in increased thirst and urine production. However, in the normal state, the actions of insulin prevent blood sugar concentrations from exceeding the renal threshold.

Type 1 diabetes mellitus box 2

Case note: Diagnosis

How does an understanding of glucose and insulin physiology allow the diagnosis to be made so rapidly?

The rapid diagnosis was based on the testing of the urine for glucose and ketones. Glucose is normally filtered through the glomerular membrane of the kidney and is nearly all reabsorbed at the proximal tubule. However, the capacity for resorption is limited. When high serum glucose levels exceed the capacity of the kidney (this varies but is at a concentration of approximately 10 mmol/L, or 180 mg/dL), glucose appears in the urine (glycosuria). This is easily detected by testing the urine with a dipstick. The detection of glycosuria

by the nurse fitted with the finding of ketones in the urine and the clinical situation: young age, weight loss and symptoms of tiredness, passing a lot of urine (polyuria) and considerable thirst with high fluid intake (polydipsia). This led the doctor immediately to diagnose insulin-dependent diabetes mellitus.

The presence of glucose in the urine causes an osmotic diuresis. This is the reason for dehydration and thirst. Unfortunately, Robert's attempts to quench his thirst with soft drinks actually worsened the situation. This is because most soft drinks contain high levels of glucose.

Insulin and the response to high blood glucose levels

Anatomy of the pancreas

The pancreas is an abdominal organ, with its head lying in the C-curve of the duodenum (Fig. 9.3). The

pancreas is a lobed structure made up of the alveoli of secretory cells which drain into the large duct that runs the length of the pancreas and drains into the duodenum. The islets of Langerhans lie between the alveoli. The blood supply to the pancreas is from the splenic artery and the pancreato-duodenal artery, and venous drainage is into the portal vein. The pancreas develops from two buds off the duodenum, which migrate to join together.

The endocrine pancreas

The pancreas has two main functions: it produces digestive enzymes that are secreted directly into the duodenum (exocrine function), and hormones (endocrine function). The hormones are produced by the cells of the islets of Langerhans (Fig. 9.4), which comprise only about 2% of the mass of the pancreas. Islets are composed of four main cell types which have two different naming systems, a Greek and a Roman lettering system. The commonest are the β cells (B cells), which secrete insulin, whereas α cells (A cells) produce glucagon, and the less numerous δ cells (D cells) and PP cells (also called F cells) secrete pancreatic polypeptide (Table 9.2).

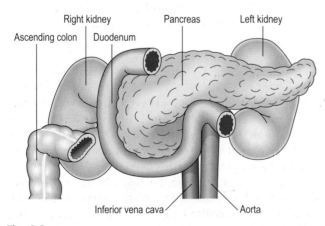

Right kidney Pancreas Left kidney
Ascending colon Duodenum
Inferior vena cava Aorta

Fig. 9.3
Anatomical location of the pancreas. Not shown are the liver and stomach; the pancreas lies behind these organs. IVC, inferior vena cava.

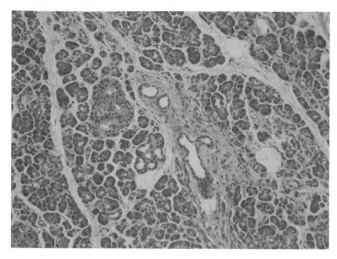

Fig. 9.4
Histological appearance of the islet of Langerhans.
(Courtesy of Dr Daniel Berney.)

Table 9.2
Cell types in the islets of Langerhans

Cell type	Alternative name	Percentage of the islet	Hormone secreted
A cell	α cell	10	Glucagon
B cell	β cell	60–80	Insulin
D cell	δ cell	~5	Somatostatin
F cell	PP cell	Varies	Pancreatic polypeptide

In insulin-dependent (type 1) diabetes there is usually immune-mediated destruction of the islets of Langerhans, resulting in severely reduced insulin secretion.

Synthesis and secretion of insulin

Insulin is a two-chain polypeptide hormone which is made from a single large precursor called pre-pro-insulin. This precursor is made in the rough endoplasmic reticulum of β cells where its pre-peptide is removed, and the protein is folded and held in place with disulphide bridges (Fig. 9.5) between the A and B chains. The resulting pro-insulin is transported to the Golgi complex where the peptide is packaged into secretory vesicles for final processing and secretion. In order to make mature insulin, the link between the A and B chains is removed by proteolysis. This linking section is called C-peptide and is secreted with insulin into the circulation, when the secretory vesicles fuse with the plasma membrane in response to an appropriate signal.

Regulation of insulin secretion

The most important stimulus to insulin secretion is an increase in the plasma glucose concentration. This is detected by a glucose transporter protein called GLUT2 (pronounced gloot two), located on the islet cells, in combination with glucokinase, which together are considered to be a glucose receptor. The GLUT2 allows entry of glucose into the β cell. The glucokinase converts glucose to glucose 6-phosphate, which is the starting point for glucose metabolism. The net result of glucose metabolism in β cells is an increase in intracellular ATP levels; this blocks ATP-sensitive potassium channels, resulting in depolarization of the cell and causing an influx of calcium through voltage-gated calcium channels. The increased intracellular calcium concentration activates calcium–calmodulin-dependent protein kinase, and leads to insulin secretion by exocytosis (Fig. 9.6).

Several other agents stimulate insulin release, including acetylcholine, bombesin, glucagon-like peptide 1 (GLP1), glucagon, cholecystokinin and glucose-dependent insulinotropic peptide (GIP), whereas adrenaline, galanin and somatostatin inhibit insulin release. Daily insulin secretion represents approximately 15% of the insulin stored in the pancreas at any time.

Insulin in blood

There is no specific carrier protein for insulin in plasma so it has a very short half-life of around 3–5 minutes. Insulin is metabolized by proteases in many tissues, principally the liver. The normal fasting insulin level is kept within a tight range and is dependent on the level of the fasting glucose. Usually for a fasting glucose level of about 5 mmol/L, the insulin ranges between 5 and 10 mU/L (35–70 pmol/L), with some variation depending on the insulin assay manufacturer.

What does insulin do?

Insulin is essential in the body as it allows cells to take up and then metabolize glucose. Without insulin the body cannot effectively handle a glucose load, such as a meal. In the absence of insulin, plasma glucose concentrations may be high but the cells of the body are effectively glucose deprived as the glucose cannot get into the cells. In most cells insulin exerts its effect by increasing the activity of a glucose transporter protein, GLUT4 (pronounced gloot four), at the plasma membrane, allowing effective uptake of glucose by the cell. In the liver, however, insulin does not affect GLUT4, but instead increases the expression of glucokinase,

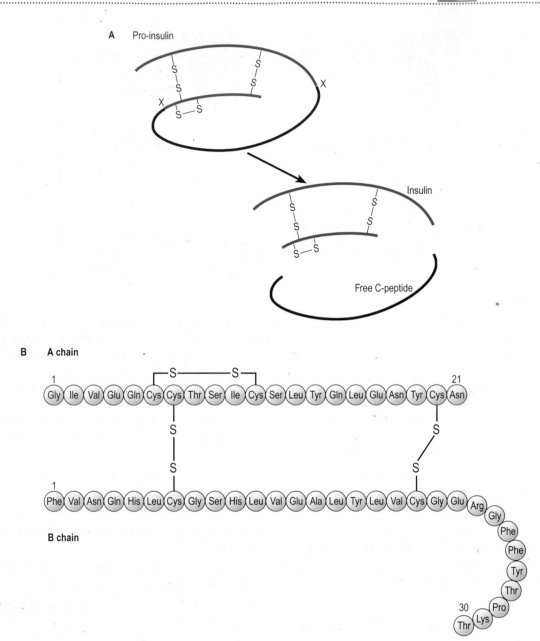

Fig. 9.5
Structure of insulin. (A) Insulin is made as part of a larger peptide molecule called pro-insulin. The action of proteases (shown by X in the diagram) cleaves the pro-insulin to give the mature insulin and free C-peptide, or connecting peptide. S–S indicate the disulphide bridges that hold the two peptide chains of insulin together. (B) Peptide sequence of human insulin.

an enzyme that phosphorylates glucose prior to its conversion to glycogen.

The net effect of insulin action is to lower blood glucose by stimulating cells to take up glucose and convert it to glycogen. However, insulin has important effects on protein and fat metabolism in addition to its effects on glucose. The metabolic effects of insulin are summarized in Box 9.1. The glucose and insulin response to food intake is shown in Figure 9.7.

The insulin receptor

Insulin is a large peptide that cannot readily enter cells. It therefore exerts its effects by binding to a receptor in the plasma membrane of its target cells. The insulin receptor consists of four subunits, two α and two β (Fig. 9.8). Insulin binds to the α subunits, causing the protein kinase domains of the β subunits to become active and initiate a phosphorylation cascade, starting with insulin

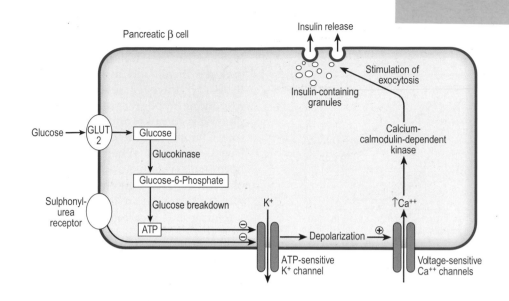

Fig. 9.6

Mechanism of glucose-stimulated insulin secretion. Glucose enters the pancreatic β cell through the GLUT2 transporter. Inside the cell the glucose is converted to glucose 6-phosphate, then broken down to yield adenosine triphosphate (ATP). The ATP causes ATP-sensitive potassium channels to close, resulting in depolarization of the cell, which causes the voltage-sensitive calcium channels to open. The resulting increase in intracellular calcium concentration activates a calcium–calmodulin-dependent kinase, stimulating exocytosis of insulin-containing granules. This exocytosis is the mechanism by which insulin is released into the blood. One of the key treatments for type 2 diabetes mellitus is a class of drugs called sulphonylureas. These act directly on a sulphonylurea receptor on the β cell and have the same effect as an increased ATP concentration: closing the potassium channels and ultimately causing an increase in insulin release.

Box 9.1

Metabolic effects of insulin

Insulin is required to maintain all of these metabolic processes. In the absence of insulin these mechanisms effectively go into reverse, an effect that is further increased by the actions of glucagon.

Effects on glucose metabolism: promotes uptake and storage of glucose

- In muscle – increases glucose uptake by cells, increases glycogen synthesis

- In liver – increases glycogen synthesis both by stimulating glycogen formation and by inhibiting glycogen breakdown (glycogenolysis)

Effects on protein metabolism: promotes protein formation

- In muscle – increases uptake of amino acids and promotes protein synthesis

- In liver – inhibits breakdown of amino acids to form glucose

Effects on fat metabolism: promotes fat storage

- In adipose tissue – increases storage of triglycerides by inducing lipoprotein lipase and inhibiting intracellular lipase. Increases esterification and storage of fatty acids

- In liver – inhibits breakdown of fatty acids to ketones. Increases synthesis of triglycerides and very low-density lipoproteins

---

receptor substrate (IRS). One of the main effects of the action of insulin is an increase in the number of GLUT4 receptors at the cell surface, so acting to increase the capacity of the cell for the uptake of glucose. For more details of insulin receptors see Chapter 1.

Glucagon and other hormones that act to raise blood glucose levels

Although insulin is the only hormone responsible for preventing blood glucose levels from rising too high,

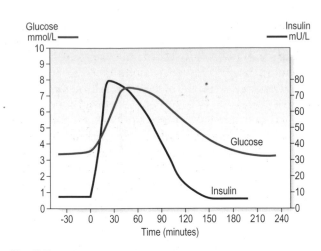

Fig. 9.7

Plasma insulin and glucose levels following a meal. Levels of both glucose and insulin increase rapidly after a meal (time 0). The time taken for values to return to fasting levels depends on both the size and nutrient composition of the meal.

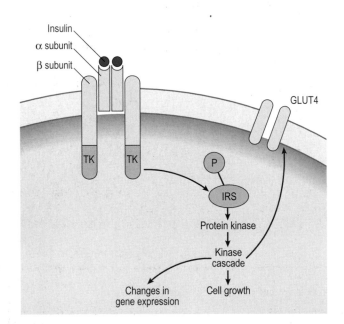

Fig. 9.8

Insulin receptor and intracellular signalling. When insulin binds to the α subunit of the receptor it causes the tyrosine kinase (TK) domain of the β subunit to become active. This results in the phosphorylation (P) of intracellular proteins, starting with the insulin receptor substrate (IRS) family. The actions of insulin lead to an increased number of GLUT4 glucose transport proteins at the cell membrane.

several hormones are involved in preventing blood glucose from falling too low. This 'multifactorial' regulation clearly reflects the importance of preventing blood glucose from becoming too low.

Classically, glucagon is the hormone that opposes the effects of insulin, and acts to raise blood glucose levels when they fall, thus maintaining blood glucose between meals and in the fasting state (see Fig. 9.2). In reality, however, several hormones act together to respond to hypoglycaemia; the maintenance of fasting glucose is complex and also involves growth hormone (see Chapter 3), catecholamines and glucocorticoids (see Chapter 4). When there are disorders of these hormonal systems, such as excess growth hormone or cortisol secretion, hyperglycaemia and impaired glucose tolerance are often seen.

Glucagon is secreted by the α cells of the pancreatic islet as a 29-amino-acid peptide. Its release is inhibited by glucose and so it is secreted in response to low glucose levels in the α cells. The effects of glucagon are mainly on the liver, where it increases the rate of glycogen breakdown (glycogenolysis) and stimulates pathways of glucose formation from amino acids (gluconeogenesis). The net effect of these actions is to raise blood glucose levels. Glucagon also acts on adipose tissue to stimulate lipolysis, the breakdown of fat stores, producing increased plasma free fatty acid concentrations. In insulin deficiency (see below) the actions of glucagon contribute significantly to the hyperglycaemia and ketosis.

Type 1 diabetes mellitus box 3

Case note: Weight loss

Why did Robert lose weight despite eating normally?

Robert lost weight because glucagon and the other glucose-mobilizing hormones were responding to the lack of glucose available to cells by working to raise plasma glucose levels. These hormones act by increasing catabolism of lipids and proteins in the body, hence reducing body fat and protein stores and causing the weight loss.

Disorders of blood glucose regulation

Type 1 diabetes: insulin deficiency (insulin-dependent diabetes mellitus)

This is a disorder that is usually first seen in young people. The cause of insulin deficiency is the destruction of β cells in the pancreatic islets. By the time diabetes mellitus has developed, most patients will have no β cells left intact. This is probably the end result of a chain of events. There may be a genetic predisposition to type 1 diabetes, and there is some link

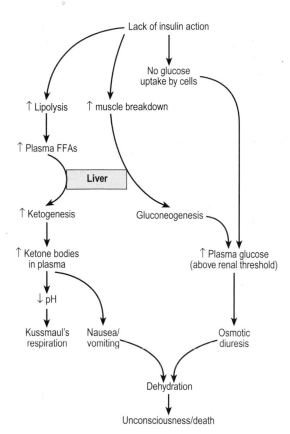

Fig. 9.9

Development of ketoacidosis. Lack of insulin action means that cells cannot use the glucose in the blood, so need to get fuel from another source. The increased level of glucagon and other hormones stimulates muscle and fat breakdown, causing a rise in plasma free fatty acids (FFAs) and a further increase in blood glucose (from glucogenic amino acids). The use of fatty acids as fuel results in the production of ketone bodies in plasma. These have two effects: lowering of blood pH (the acidosis), and nausea and vomiting. The high blood glucose level exceeds the renal threshold and causes an osmotic diuresis. Together with the nausea and vomiting, this diuresis causes dehydration, which may be life threatening. The acidosis results in Kussmaul's respiration: a deep sighing pattern of breathing in a physiological attempt to raise the blood pH by expiring as much carbon dioxide as possible.

to the human leucocyte antigen (HLA) genes. However, it is very likely that an environmental challenge (possibly viral) is needed. This leads to inflammation of the islets (called insulitis) and changes the nature of the β cell so that it becomes a target of attack by the immune system. Auto-antibodies may be detected in the serum of patients with type 1 diabetes. These antibodies are associated with β-cell destruction.

As a result of the lack of insulin, blood glucose levels are raised both after a meal and in the fasting state. As

cells have a poor uptake of glucose in the absence of insulin, they cannot 'see' the glucose in the blood, and the body responds as if it was in a state of hypoglycaemia. Sometimes diabetes mellitus is referred to as 'starvation in the midst of plenty'. All of the regulatory mechanisms for correcting hypoglycaemia are activated, so there is increased lipolysis, resulting in an increase in plasma free fatty acids, with an increased production of ketone bodies, leading to the development of ketoacidosis (Fig. 9.9). This metabolic acidosis is partly compensated by a respiratory mechanism, called 'Kussmaul's respiration', in which there is an increased rate of deep breathing. This has the effect of causing greater total expiration of carbon dioxide, and so reduces the level of dissolved carbon dioxide in the blood, raising the pH of the blood.

Type 1 diabetes mellitus box 4

Case note: Investigations

The doctor at the health centre arranged for Robert's admission and treatment with insulin. The blood tests showed:

Plasma glucose	22 mmol/L (normal fasting 3–6 mmol/L)
Plasma insulin	<5 mU/L (normal fasting 5–10 mU/L)
Anti-pancreatic islet cell antibodies	220 kU/L (normal <60 kU/L)

How does an understanding of pathology and immunology explain these results?

Interesting fact

Diabetes was described in ancient Egyptian and Greek medical texts, but it was not until the end of the 19th century that the role of the pancreas was realized. Removal of the pancreas in dogs resulted in diabetes but, puzzlingly, injection of an extract of whole pancreas did not reverse the condition. We now know that this is because the insulin was broken down by proteolytic enzymes from the exocrine part of the pancreas.

It was Frederick Banting who in 1921 deduced that this problem might be overcome by ligating the blood supply to the pancreas in dogs, waiting for 6 weeks for the exocrine pancreas to die off, then producing an extract from the remaining pancreas. At the time, Banting's medical practice was not particularly successful so he took a job as a physiology demonstrator at the University of Ontario to pay the bills. He was unable to convince his head of department, John McLeod, of the value of the proposed experiment, but was eventually given a disused laboratory, a medical student (Charles Best) as an assistant, and 2 months to test his theory. The first ligatures were unsuccessful, but McLeod agreed to an extension of the project, which Banting sold his car to finance, and the rest is history.

Type 1 diabetes mellitus box 5

Case note: Explanation

How does an understanding of pathology and immunology explain these results?

The presence of high levels of anti-pancreatic islet cell antibodies shows that Robert's diabetes is associated with an immune-mediated destruction of the pancreatic islet cells, causing loss of insulin production. It is thought that an environmental event triggers the autoimmune attack in individuals with a genetic vulnerability. Certain genetic variants in the histocompatibility (HLA) loci on the short arm of chromosome 6 give a high risk of type 1 diabetes mellitus. The environmental triggers include infections (particularly enteroviruses). An immune response includes activated T lymphocytes and macrophages, which are found invading the pancreatic islets. Autoantibodies may become detectable in the serum, well before the onset of clinical diabetes mellitus. These antibodies are targeted to islet cells, insulin, glutamate decarboxylase and insulinoma-related antigen 2. Islet cell antibodies predict a risk of future type 1 diabetes mellitus of 20–30%, compared with a general population risk of about 1 in 400 (0.25%).

Type 2 diabetes (non-insulin-dependent diabetes)

In this disorder there is usually normal or raised insulin secretion, but also a degree of insulin receptor insensitivity. This means that higher levels of insulin are required to achieve the same effect. It is therefore a disorder of *relative* insulin deficiency. Type 2 diabetes is far more common than type 1 diabetes, and is more likely to be seen in obese individuals. There are several factors that appear to contribute to the disorder,

including a strong genetic component, but the underlying mechanism leading to type 2 diabetes is not well understood. It is possible that type 2 diabetes is a group of closely related disorders, including the 'metabolic syndrome', that share the common feature of relative insulin deficiency (see section on the Metabolic syndrome below).

The result of the insulin resistance is that high levels of insulin secretion are required to maintain normal blood glucose levels. In many individuals this high rate of secretion is not sustainable and β-cell function progressively declines, with some people ultimately requiring insulin treatment to maintain glycaemic control.

The oral glucose tolerance test

An oral glucose tolerance test (Fig. 9.10) may be used to confirm a diagnosis of diabetes mellitus, although it is more usual simply to measure fasting blood glucose and free fatty acids. The test is based on measuring how the body deals with a glucose load. The person fasts overnight and in the morning is given a fixed dose of glucose, usually in the form of a sweet drink. Blood samples are taken at 30-minute intervals for 2 hours, and both glucose and insulin concentrations are measured.

Type 1 diabetes mellitus box 6

Case note: Glycaemic control

Some 6 months later Robert collapsed while out at a pub with friends. He was taken by ambulance to the accident and emergency department, where he was admitted to the hospital.

He recovered after treatment, but was very frightened by the experience.

Why did he collapse?

Following his hospital admission, Robert was given an appointment in the diabetes clinic. A blood sample was taken and the results showed an HbA1c measurement of 8.3% (normal range 4.5–6.0%).

Robert was advised to monitor his blood glucose more frequently, and was referred to the diabetes nurse for advice on diet and lifestyle. He was warned of the consequences of poor long-term glycaemic control.

What is HbA1c and what is the significance of a high reading?

What are the long-term consequences of poor glycaemic control?

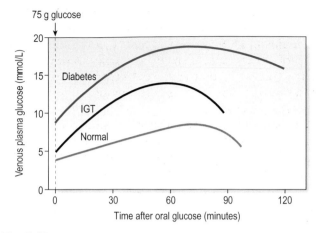

75 g glucose

Fig. 9.10
Normal and abnormal oral glucose tolerance test results.
The figure also shows 'impaired glucose tolerance' (IGT)
in a person who is developing diabetes.

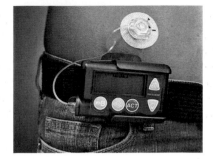

Fig. 9.11
An insulin pump. (Reproduced from Chew S L, Leslie D
2006 Clinical endocrinology and diabetes: an illustrated
colour text. Churchill Livingstone, Edinburgh.)

Management of diabetes mellitus

A key aspect of the management of both type 1 and
type 2 diabetes is diet. The aim is to avoid a rapid rise
in circulating glucose levels. So the advice given is to
avoid foods containing simple carbohydrates (such as
sucrose – normal 'sugar') and to eat regular meals containing complex carbohydrates such as bread, pasta
and potatoes. This produces a slow release of glucose from the digestive tract into the blood and can
help avoid periods of excessively high blood glucose.
Diabetes is also associated with high serum lipid concentrations, which are linked to cardiovascular disease, so people with diabetes are also advised to avoid
fatty foods and to increase consumption of cereals,
fruit and vegetables.

Type 2 diabetes may be managed by dietary control alone, especially if there is a return to 'normal'
weight. However, compliance with dietary advice is
often poor.

Drug treatment of type 2 diabetes

There are two main groups of drugs used to treat
type 2 diabetes: one group acts to increase the release
of insulin from the pancreas and the other group acts
to enhance the actions of insulin on target cells. The
first group of drugs are called the sulphonylureas.
They bind to specific receptors on β cells, causing
the closure of potassium channels and resulting in
depolarization of the cell, calcium entry and release of
insulin (see Fig. 9.6). It might seem obvious, but these
drugs are effective only when pancreatic β cells are
intact and functional.

The second group of drugs are the biguanides, the
best known of which is metformin. These drugs do not
require functional β cells in order to be effective. Their
exact mechanism of action is not clear but they appear
to exert several different effects, causing a decrease
in hepatic gluconeogenesis, increased uptake of glucose by peripheral muscle cells and decreased intestinal glucose absorbance. Taken together, these actions
result in a lowering of blood glucose concentrations.

Insulin therapy

For patients with type 1 diabetes, and also patients
with type 2 diabetes who no longer have functional
pancreatic β cells, treatment with insulin is required.
Insulin is a large peptide hormone, so it is not orally
active and must therefore be injected regularly. Various
preparations are available, ranging from short acting
to very long acting. Regular blood glucose monitoring
is essential for people on insulin treatment. In patients
given insulin for diabetic ketoacidosis, serum potassium levels fall quickly and serum potassium should
be monitored and supplements given. This is because
the action of insulin causes potassium to shift into cells
with glucose. A relatively new development in insulin therapy is the use of insulin pumps, which deliver
a continuous infusion of insulin subcutaneously
(Fig. 9.11). These are particularly useful in people
who find it difficult to achieve good control of blood
glucose using other methods.

Measurement of blood glucose
At home
As the main aim in the management of diabetes mellitus is to enable the person to maintain normal blood
glucose levels, it is important to have a simple method
for measuring these levels that the patient can use at
home and at work. Pocket-sized glucose monitors are
widely available and give an accurate reading from a
finger-prick blood sample (Fig. 9.12). People with type
1 diabetes are advised to check their blood glucose

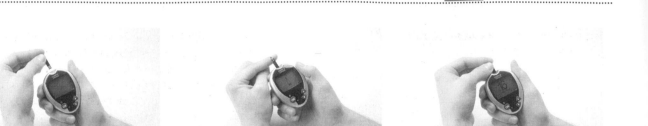

Fig. 9.12
A home test meter for blood glucose level. (A) A new test strip is placed in the meter. (B) A drop of blood is applied to the strip. (C) After a few seconds, the blood glucose level appears on the meter screen. OneTouch® Ultra® is a registered trademark of LifeScan Inc. (Image courtesy of LifeScan Inc.)

four to five times a day – more frequently if they are unwell or under stress. People with type 2 diabetes are generally advised to check less regularly as large fluctuations in blood glucose levels are less usual in type 2 diabetes.

Regular testing is generally thought to improve glycaemic control and lead to fewer long-term complications. This is partly because the patient can take appropriate action if the level is too low or too high, but also because monitoring glucose levels regularly allows the patient to learn the consequences of missing meals, eating cakes, etc.

In the diabetes clinic
Home blood glucose monitoring gives a useful 'snapshot' of the glucose concentration at that moment, but it is useful for a physician to get a picture of how well the patient is controlling their blood glucose over a longer period of time. The best measure of this is the glycated haemoglobin concentration (HbA1c).

Haemoglobin in red blood cells naturally forms a complex with glucose. The amount of the complex formed is directly proportional to the concentration of glucose in the blood. Thus, measuring the proportion of haemoglobin that is glycated gives an indication of 'average' blood glucose levels. As red blood cells have a life of 120 days, the reading indicates how well blood glucose was controlled over the last couple of months. A high reading suggests that blood glucose has not been well controlled and the aim is to keep HbA1c as close to the normal range (4.5–6.0%) as possible.

Type 1 diabetes mellitus box 7

Case note: Explanation

It is likely that Robert collapsed because he was not eating regularly. He would have been prescribed insulin in two forms: a long-acting and short-acting form. The long-acting form is used to regulate blood glucose between meals, and the short-acting form is used at meal times. If somebody using the long-acting form does not eat regularly, they may become hypoglycaemic and collapse. The chances of this happening are increased by the consumption of alcohol.

Short-term complications of diabetes mellitus

Diabetic ketoacidosis
Ketoacidosis may be the first presentation of diabetes. There is hyperglycaemia, with nausea, and a characteristic sweet smell to the breath. See Figure 9.9 for an explanation of the development of ketoacidosis. Kussmaul's respiration is a deep sighing breathing that develops in an attempt to compensate for the decreased pH. Deeper breathing decreases the partial pressure of carbon dioxide ($P\text{co}_2$), which causes a rise in pH.

Hypoglycaemic coma
This is usually the result of taking insulin but not eating enough to maintain blood glucose levels. Blood sugar concentration is very low. This is a life-threatening condition that must be treated promptly. Many diabetics can tell when they are about to become hypoglycaemic and carry a sweet to eat in emergencies.

Long-term consequences of poor glycaemic control

The chronic complications of diabetes mellitus are very clearly linked to the effectiveness of glycaemic control (Fig. 9.13). With good control of blood glucose these complications may be delayed indefinitely. Most of the complications arise from damage to small blood vessels. The effects of this include diabetic retinopathy and nephropathy, and may also result, in extreme cases, in gangrene.

There are also effects on large blood vessels that appear to mirror an acceleration of atherosclerosis, causing increased incidence of myocardial infarction and stroke. In addition, poor glycaemic control is associated with a peripheral neuropathy particularly affecting sensory nerves, resulting in tingling, itching and other abnormal sensory perceptions.

There is also an increased incidence of infection and poor wound healing.

Type 2 diabetes mellitus box 8

Case note: Action of insulin

How does an understanding of the action of insulin explain the ketosis and ketonuria observed at Robert's initial presentation?

Insulin is anabolic and produces polymers and macromolecules, such as glycogen and protein, from smaller molecules, such as glucose and amino acids (see Box 9.1). It allows glucose to be used by the different cells in the body. If insulin is absent, cells cannot take up glucose efficiently, so the body 'looks for' another source of energy. In the absence of insulin, fat stores break down and release free fatty acids, which are in turn broken down into ketones. The combination of ketonuria and glycosuria strongly suggests insulin-dependent diabetes mellitus. The breakdown of glycogen to glucose, and of protein to amino acids, also contributes to weight loss and wasting of muscle.

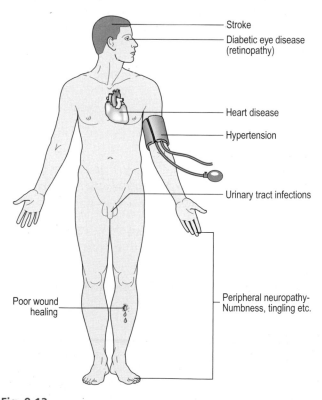

Fig. 9.13
Complications of poor control of blood glucose in diabetes mellitus.

The metabolic syndrome – a growing problem?

Most people in the developed world, if they have any interest in current affairs, will know of the serious concerns about the 'obesity epidemic' sweeping the USA and Europe. This concern is reflected in government advice on healthy eating, exercise and in the 'Healthy Schools' programme of the British Government in 2005. As a general rule, we are consuming more calories than we need and becoming seriously overweight. This is causing serious health problems in the

---

Interesting fact

The metabolic syndrome is not a new concept. It can be recognized in classical clinical descriptions from the 19th century. For example, Samuel Gee, a physician at St Bartholomew's Hospital from 1866 to 1904, wrote:

'there is a diathesis which is very common, but for which it is difficult to find an appropriate name, because we do not understand its nature or essence. Among the diseases related to or dependent upon this diathesis are gout, gravel, obesity, diabetes, granular kidneys and arterio-capillary sclerosis.'

populations of the richest countries, including an increase in a condition known as the 'metabolic syndrome'. This syndrome is a combination of common diseases that confer an increased risk of future vascular disease and type 2 diabetes mellitus. It has recently been estimated that 25% of all adult Americans have this syndrome. However, the metabolic syndrome is not simply a result of over-eating. It is also associated with other disorders, particularly schizophrenia, where there is a twofold to fourfold increased risk of developing the metabolic syndrome compared with that in the general population.

Diagnosis of the metabolic syndrome

The key components of the syndrome are central or abdominal obesity, insulin resistance, hypertension and dyslipidaemia (Fig. 9.14). A set of 'typical' blood test results is shown in Box 9.2. The clinical usefulness of defining a metabolic syndrome is still controversial and the condition has several other names (syndrome X, Reaven's syndrome or insulin resistance syndrome). A particular controversy is whether the combination of diseases carries a greater risk than the sum of the risks of the individual diseases. One major clinical benefit in considering the metabolic syndrome is that if one feature is found then the others should be sought.

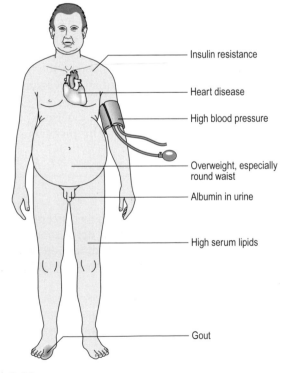

Fig. 9.14
Person with the metabolic syndrome.

Different criteria are used for its diagnosis, depending on the sponsoring organization. The criteria from the World Health Organization are shown in Box 9.3. The lack of a single consensus set of diagnostic criteria means that estimates of the prevalence of the metabolic syndrome vary, but most studies are in agreement that the prevalence in the developed world is increasing rapidly. Smoking has a further impact on

---

Box 9.2

Typical fasting blood tests in a patient with the metabolic syndrome

Glucose	6.8 mmol/L (normal 3–5 mmol/L)
Insulin	34 mU/L (normal <10 mU/L)
Total cholesterol	7.9 mmol/L (normal <5.0 mmol/L)
LDL-cholesterol	4.3 mmol/L (normal <3.0 mmol/L)
HDL-cholesterol	0.8 mmol/L (normal >1.15 mmol/L)
Triglycerides	5.1 mmol/L (normal <1.5 mmol/L)
Urine albumin: creatinine ratio	40 mg/g (normal <30 mg/g)

The key points here are: raised fasting glucose indicating insulin resistance; raised total cholesterol and low-density lipoprotein (LDL)-cholesterol with reduced high-density lipoprotein (HDL)-cholesterol, demonstrating dyslipidaemia; and a raised urine albumin:creatinine ratio, indicating early renal disease, probably as a result of hypertension.

Box 9.3

Diagnostic criteria for the metabolic syndrome as defined by the World Health Organization

Diabetes/impaired fasting glucose/impaired glucose tolerance/insulin resistance *and* at least two of the following criteria:

① Waist:hip ratio >0.90 in men and >0.85 in women (central obesity)

② Serum triglycerides >1.7 mmol/L *or* HDL-cholesterol <0.9 mmol/L in men and <1.0 mmol/L in women

③ Blood pressure >140/90 mmHg

④ Urinary albumin excretion rate >20 μg/min *or* albumin:creatinine ratio >30 mg/g

increasing vascular disease but is not included in most diagnostic criteria.

The first description of the metabolic syndrome?

Samuel Gee described a case of a man in his forties who was 'robust, even sporty' in his youth, but who has now gone to seed, drinking a bottle of claret a day, eating in expensive restaurants and smoking cigarettes. He has become obese with a flushed complexion, impaired glucose tolerance and hypertension. This cautionary tale concludes with the reprobate refusing to comply with his doctor's advice to change his lifestyle and, as a result, dying from a cerebral haemorrhage. (Adapted from Samuel Gee 1908 *Medical Lectures and Aphorisms*. Henry Frowde Hodder & Stoughton, London, Chapter 1.)

How is the metabolic syndrome treated?

We now know that the metabolic syndrome is not caused just by a surfeit of claret, and the clinical approach to the metabolic syndrome involves the aggressive treatment of each component. A diet and exercise programme benefits most patients, who should be advised to keep alcohol intake to a minimum. However, compliance with lifestyle changes is generally poor and most patients will require drugs to control lipid levels and blood pressure.

The lipids can be controlled with an HMG CoA (3-hydroxy-3-methylglutaryl coenzyme A) reductase inhibitor (a statin), which lowers low-density lipoprotein-cholesterol levels and raises high-density lipoprotein-cholesterol levels. The hypertension is usually treated with either an angiotensin converting enzyme (ACE) inhibitor or an angiotensin-2 receptor antagonist. This treatment both lowers blood pressure and reduces albuminuria.

There may be benefit in prescribing metformin (a drug that sensitizes the cells to insulin action) in addition to the other treatments. Metformin is a biguanide that has several effects on glucose metabolism. It reduces the production of glucose by the liver and increases the uptake and oxidation of glucose by skeletal muscle. There may also be a modest weight loss with metformin treatment. However, 'lifestyle counselling' remains the key to decreasing both the prevalence and the consequences of this very modern disease.

Self-assessment case study

A case of coma

Rosie Brown was 19 years old and was brought to the hospital because of unconsciousness. The history was obtained from her friends and the ambulance crew. She had apparently been well, but very quiet, the previous day and had gone to bed after a night out with her friends. She did not come down for breakfast and a friend went into her room to wake her and found her unresponsive, pale and clammy. The ambulance was called and the crew reported shallow breathing and a faint fast pulse. The blood pressure was 85/30 mmHg. She was given oxygen by mask and an intravenous line was inserted. A drop of blood was tested with a portable glucose monitor and the blood sugar level was 0.5 mmol/L. She was immediately given 50 mL 50% dextrose intravenously and glucagon 1 mg intramuscularly.

Ms Brown had been fit and well previously. She was on the oral contraceptive pill and consumed about two glasses of wine a night. She was a student nurse and shared the house with three other students.

On examination, she looked drowsy. Her skin was cold and clammy. She was not able to respond coherently to questions, but was able to obey simple commands to open her eyes and move her limbs. Her pulse was 120 beats per minute in sinus tachycardia and her blood pressure was 110/70 mmHg. There were no other abnormal clinical signs.

The finger-prick blood glucose level was 2.2 mmol/L and further blood samples were taken. A further injection of 50% glucose was given, followed by a dextrose infusion. Her consciousness level and confusion improved over the next 12 hours.

The laboratory tests showed:

Plasma glucose	2.0 mmol/L (normal 4.0–6.0 mmol/L)
Serum insulin	930 pmol/L (normal 35–140 pmol/L)
Serum C-peptide	<0.5 nmol/L (normal 0.5–1.15 nmol/L)
Urine sulphonylurea	Negative

Questions:

① How does knowledge of endogenous insulin production help in the interpretation of her biochemical investigations?

② What is the likeliest diagnosis?

③ Her dextrose infusion is stopped at 12 hours, but her confusion returns. What is the likeliest diagnosis?

④ What is the purpose of the urine sulphonylurea test?

Answers see page 149

Extended matching questions

A   Diathesis
B   Exocytosis
C   Gluconeogenesis
D   Glycation of haemoglobin
E   Glycogenolysis
F   Glycosuria
G   Insulin resistance
H   Ketoacidosis
I   Lipolysis
J   Osmotic diuresis
K   Phosphorylation cascade
L   Proteolysis

For each of the definitions below, select the most appropriate term from the list above:

① This process is initiated by insulin binding to the α subunit of its receptor and activating the protein tyrosine kinase domains of the β subunits.

② This process allows a simple test indicating average blood sugar levels over a period of time.

③ The process by which mature insulin is formed from its precursor, pro-insulin.

④ The process by which insulin is released from islet cells.

⑤ This process is inhibited in the liver by the actions of insulin.

⑥ This process is stimulated in fat stores by the actions of glucagon.

Answers see page 153

HORMONAL REGULATION OF PLASMA CALCIUM AND CALCIUM METABOLISM

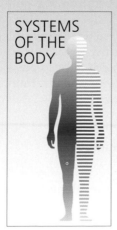

SYSTEMS
OF THE
BODY

Chapter objectives

After reading this chapter you should be able to:

① Understand the significance of maintaining plasma calcium levels.

② Understand the hormonal regulation of plasma calcium.

③ Appreciate the interactions between parathyroid hormone and vitamin D3.

④ Understand the regulation of parathyroid hormone secretion.

⑤ Appreciate the significance of renal function in calcium metabolism.

⑥ Have an understanding of disorders of calcium metabolism and metabolic bone disease.

Introduction

Calcium is a metal ion that is widespread in the body and has a wide range of functions. It is an important component of intracellular signalling pathways (see Chapter 1). It is also necessary for the activity of some enzymes and for the binding of hormones to receptors. An appropriate level of calcium is required for nerve transmission at the neuromuscular junction. However, most of the calcium within the body is stored in the skeleton, complexed with phosphate.

Interesting fact

Calcium accounts for 1.5–2% of adult body weight, so that the average person contains between 1 and 1.5 kg of elemental calcium, mostly in bone.

Primary hyperparathyroidism box 1

Case history

Joan Smith was 65 years old. She had become very tired over many months, if not years. The symptoms were so insidious in onset that she could not remember when they began with any precision. She had passed urine three or four times a night for several years. In the past year she had become very constipated, passing hard stools only once or twice a week. In the last few weeks she had also been feeling nauseous.

The past history included an episode of renal colic about 15 years previously. Mrs Smith had passed the stone in her urine.

On examination she appeared fatigued and low in mood. Her blood pressure was 165/95 mmHg. There were several mobile lumps in the abdomen which were thought to be hard faeces in the colon. The rectum contained hard faeces.

Serum calcium

Serum calcium concentrations are maintained within a very tight range. The normal serum calcium concentration is between 2.2 and 2.5 mmol/L. Approximately half of this is free, ionized calcium, and the remainder is either bound to plasma proteins or complexed, with citrate for example.

The consequences of plasma calcium straying outside these limits are significant. Hypocalcaemia results in hyperexcitability of the neuromuscular junction, leading to pins and needles, then tetany, paralysis and even convulsions, whereas chronic hypercalcaemia may result in the formation of kidney stones (renal calculi), constipation, dehydration, kidney damage, tiredness and depression.

Primary hyperparathyroidism box 2

Case note: Investigations

Mrs Smith has a history and symptoms that suggest chronic hypercalcaemia. Investigations were requested, including blood tests, abdominal radiography, and a urine specimen for microbiology and cytology.

Interesting fact

It is the free, ionized calcium in plasma that is physiologically active, but common laboratory tests measure total calcium, which includes that which is bound to albumin and other proteins. Increases or decreases in the levels of these plasma proteins will obviously affect the amounts of physiologically active calcium in the blood, so the total calcium is 'corrected' to take account of the albumin concentration. It is this corrected value that is used to determine whether the calcium levels are abnormal.

Sources of serum calcium

The vast bulk of the body's calcium store is stored in the skeleton. Although the skeleton is often considered to be simply structural, bone is a readily available source of calcium (Box 10.1), and will be sacrificed if necessary to maintain serum calcium levels (Fig. 10.1). Calcium is also actively resorbed in the kidney, and dietary calcium is absorbed from the gut. This latter source is the only mechanism by which total body calcium can be increased, so it is important that this absorption occurs efficiently, especially in children and pregnant women who need to be in positive calcium balance. The availability of calcium from each of these sources is under hormonal control.

Hormones involved in the regulation of serum calcium

Given the consequences of dysregulation of serum calcium, it is clearly important that levels are maintained within set limits. Two key hormones are involved in the regulation of serum calcium concentrations: parathyroid hormone (PTH) and vitamin D. They both raise serum calcium concentrations, but act by different mechanisms and over quite different timescales. The short-term regulation of serum calcium is under the control of PTH, whereas vitamin D (calcitriol) is responsible for longer-term regulation.

Box 10.1

Bone: structure and metabolism

The adult human skeleton contains calcium complexed with phosphate to form hydroxyapatite crystals. Bone is formed by the action of cells called *osteoblasts*, which produce a collagen matrix that is mineralized with hydroxyapatite. This process is called bone deposition. The opposite effect, bone resorption, is due to the action of *osteoclasts* which generate an acidic micro-environment, causing the hydroxyapatite to dissolve, thus increasing serum calcium and phosphate levels.

Bone is a dynamic tissue which is constantly being broken down and reforming. In healthy adults the rate of bone resorption is usually equal to the rate of deposition, but under some circumstances there is a greater rate of resorption.

You can easily remember the difference between osteoblasts and osteoclasts because 'Blasts are Builders', whereas 'Clasts Claw away bone'.

Parathyroid hormone

The parathyroid glands

PTH is secreted by the chief cells of the parathyroid gland (Fig. 10.2). There are usually four parathyroid glands, located on the posterior surface of the thyroid gland. These glands are small in size, each weighing around 50 mg, but may weigh as much as 70 mg. Women usually have larger parathyroid glands than men. Embryologically, the superior and inferior pairs of parathyroid glands have different origins, although both are endodermal. The superior pair of parathyroids derive from the fourth branchial pouch and do not migrate during fetal development, while the inferior parathyroids develop from the third branchial pouch and migrate caudally to sit at the lower pole of the thyroid gland. Changes in this migratory process appear to account for the rather variable position of the lower parathyroid glands.

Interesting fact

Although there are usually four parathyroid glands, there is a great variation between individuals. One person was reported to have 104 distinct parathyroid glands, located throughout the neck region. The parathyroids are usually found attached to the thyroid gland, but may be found in other locations, including being embedded within the thyroid itself, or attached to the oesophagus.

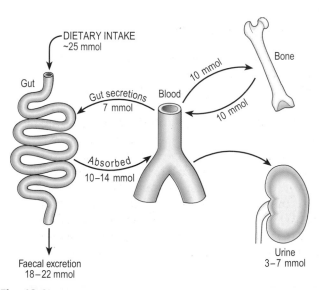

Fig. 10.1
Sources of plasma calcium. This figure shows approximate daily calcium turnover for an adult in calcium balance. It is important to recognize that calcium in bone is not all fixed, but can contribute to plasma levels of calcium.

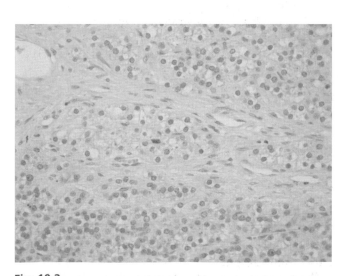

Fig. 10.2
Histology of parathyroid gland. (Courtesy of Dr Daniel Berney.)

Secretion of parathyroid hormone

PTH is a peptide hormone comprising 84 amino acids. Like many peptide hormones, it is stored within the cells and rapidly released when required. Secretion of PTH is stimulated by a low serum calcium concentration and inhibited by high serum calcium (Fig. 10.3). There are specific calcium-sensing receptors on the surface of the chief cells that monitor serum calcium levels. Phosphate may have a role in regulating PTH secretion, with high concentrations stimulating secretion, but this effect may also be a consequence of the high phosphate levels causing a reduction in serum calcium concentration. As a peptide, PTH has a very short half-life in blood of around 5 minutes.

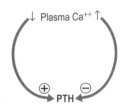

Fig. 10.3
Regulation of parathyroid hormone (PTH) secretion. This is a very simple regulatory system. Calcium sensors on the secretory cells respond to changes in plasma calcium concentrations; a low plasma calcium level stimulates PTH secretion while a high concentration is inhibitory.

Primary hyperparathyroidism box 3

Case note: Test results

The investigations revealed:

Creatinine	112 μmol/L (normal <120 μmol/L)
Serum phosphate	0.8 mmol/L (normal 0.8–1.2 mmol/L)
Albumin	42 g/L (normal 36–48 g/L)
Serum calcium	3.45 mmol/L
Corrected serum calcium	3.41 mmol/L (normal 2.2–2.6 mmol/L)
Thyroid function, electrolytes, glucose	Normal
Alkaline phosphatase	220 U/L (normal <120 U/L)
Liver function tests	Normal
Abdominal radiography	Extensive faeces throughout colon and calcification over renal areas
Urine microbiology	Normal

What other test is needed to work out what has gone wrong with calcium homeostasis?

Mrs Smith has a high serum calcium level and the main acute regulator of serum calcium homeostasis is parathyroid hormone (PTH). PTH secretion from the parathyroid glands is normally stimulated by hypocalcaemia and inhibited by hypercalcaemia. So the further investigation was to measure serum PTH, which was abnormal at 15 pmol/L (normal range 1.2–6.7 pmol/L). Because PTH should normally be inhibited by the high serum calcium concentration, this suggests that the parathyroid glands are autonomously producing excessive PTH, which has caused the hypercalcaemia. PTH causes hypercalcaemia by acting on the kidneys and bone to mobilize calcium. The high alkaline phosphatase level is a marker of bone turnover.

Actions of parathyroid hormone

The main target tissue of PTH is the kidney. PTH has two important effects in the kidney: first, to increase the reabsorption of calcium from urine, and second to increase the expression of the enzyme 1α-hydroxylase, which activates vitamin D (Fig. 10.4).

PTH, as a peptide, acts on cell surface receptors and exerts its intracellular effects by stimulating cyclic adenosine monophosphate (cAMP) production (see Chapter 1). Measurement of cAMP in urine can be used as an indication of PTH activity. PTH is a fast-acting hormone, causing a decrease in urinary calcium levels within a few minutes.

The second major target tissue for PTH is bone. PTH increases osteoclast activity, causing an increase in bone resorption.

Calcitriol: source and activation of vitamin D

There are two forms of vitamin D. The first is vitamin D3 (cholecalciferol), which can be made in the skin or derived from dietary sources such as dairy produce,

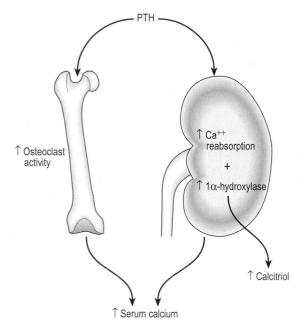

Fig. 10.4
Actions of parathyroid hormone (PTH). The target organs are bone and kidney. PTH has a rapid effect on these tissues, stimulating calcium resorption from urine and activating osteoclasts. PTH also stimulates the activation of vitamin D in the kidney.

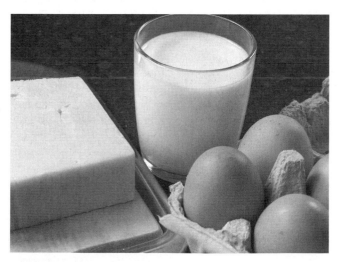

Fig. 10.5
Dietary sources of vitamin D. Dairy products (shown) are good sources of vitamin D, as are fish and some meat, particularly liver. Vitamin D is added as a supplement to margarines.

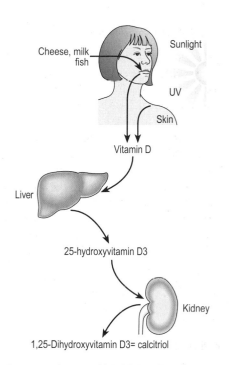

Fig. 10.6
Sources and activation of vitamin D3. Vitamin D is obtained either from the skin through the action of sunlight, or from the diet. It is relatively inactive until it has been hydroxylated twice; the first reaction takes place in the liver and the second in the kidney, leading to the formation of the active hormone, calcitriol. UV, ultraviolet light.

oily fish and liver (Fig. 10.5). The second type of vitamin D is vitamin D2 (ergocalciferol), which is derived from yeast and fungi and is added to margarines as a food supplement. Both are activated to form calcitriol, and the two forms of calcitriol are equipotent. As there is little difference between vitamins D2 and D3, they are usually just referred to as 'vitamin D'.

Calcitriol has an important role in the long-term regulation of plasma calcium levels and is made from vitamin D, a steroid derivative. Calcitriol is an unusual hormone in that it is not produced by a single gland or cell type and it is regulated in a different way from most hormones.

Vitamin D, the precursor of calcitriol, can either be obtained from the diet or made in the skin, by the action of sunlight (Fig. 10.6). The conversion of 7-dehydrocholesterol to vitamin D3 requires both light and heat. The optimal wavelength for production is 297 nm – in the ultraviolet range. Following the action of sunlight, the pre-vitamin D needs to remain in the warm skin for a while until the vitamin D is formed. So vitamin D is not really a true vitamin, as people whose skin is exposed to sufficient sunlight do not need a dietary source.

It would be very unusual if the production of a hormone were not closely regulated, and clearly the supply of vitamin D to the body is not regulated. However, both vitamin D2 and D3 are relatively inactive and

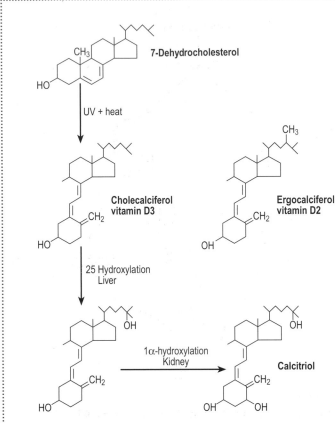

Fig. 10.7

Formation and structure of vitamin D3 (cholecalciferol) and D2 (ergocalciferol), and the formation of calcitriol. UV, ultraviolet light.

must undergo a process of chemical conversion to calcitriol in order to have significant effect (see Fig. 10.6). It is this conversion process that is actively regulated. There are two steps in the activation of vitamin D, both hydroxylation reactions. The first step is a 25-hydroxylation, which occurs in the liver and is not regulated. The second step is 1α-hydroxylation, which takes place in the kidney (Fig. 10.7). The expression of the enzyme that catalyses this reaction is actively regulated by PTH. The final active product of vitamin D activation is calcitriol.

Interesting fact

Don't be confused by the naming of this hormone, because it is known by several different names, although calcitriol is the easiest to remember. Vitamin D3 is properly known as cholecalciferol and so the active form, following the two hydroxylations, is 1,25-dihydroxycholecalciferol. It is also sometimes called 'active vitamin D3'. So 1,25-dihydroxycholecalciferol = 1,25-dihydroxyvitamin D = calcitriol. Likewise 1,25-dihydroxyergocalciferol = 1,25-dihydroxyvitamin D = calcitriol.

Vitamin D and calcitriol in blood

Vitamin D, formed in the skin or absorbed in the gut, binds to a vitamin D binding protein in blood. It has only a short half-life in blood as it is rapidly converted to 25-hydroxyvitamin D in the liver. This compound has a half-life of about 2 weeks. However, the active hormone, calcitriol, has a short half-life of just a few hours.

Actions of calcitriol

As a steroid derivative, calcitriol acts on intracellular receptors to alter the rate of transcription of certain genes. These effects are generally long-term regulatory actions. Calcitriol acts on cells in the gastrointestinal tract to increase the production of calcium transport proteins, which results in increased uptake of calcium from the gut into the body. This is the only mechanism by which the body can increase its calcium stores. Calcitriol also affects bone, increasing the rate of bone resorption and thus causing an increase in serum calcium levels. It has a minor effect on the kidney, decreasing urinary loss of calcium by stimulating reabsorption.

Interesting fact

During the Second World War, chalk (calcium carbonate) was added to all flour, and vitamin D was added to margarine in order to prevent rickets, which had been prevalent up to that time. Rickets had previously been treated (although not prevented) with cod liver oil – not very popular among the children required to take it. The staple diet of many poor, malnourished communities was bread and margarine, so these were the most obvious foods to supplement. Since that time many food laws have been passed, but all still require the supplementation of all flour with calcium carbonate, and of margarine with vitamin D.

Primary hyperparathyroidism box 4

Case note: Explanation

An understanding of calcium physiology helps in understanding the symptoms. Urinary symptoms tend to occur early in the evolution of the disease. Serum calcium is filtered in the urine and, at high levels, acts as an osmotic diuretic. Thus, in Mrs Smith, the high level of calcium in the urine increased the volume of the urine and led to nocturia. Calcium also came out of solution and formed stones. This resulted in renal colic. Hypertension was a consequence of the long exposure of the kidneys to high calcium levels.

When serum calcium levels are higher, abdominal and general symptoms occur. Calcium is important for nerve and muscle function. The muscle of the gut fails to contract properly when the calcium level is too high, resulting in constipation. Depression and tiredness are cerebral effects of high calcium levels.

Very high serum calcium levels (as in parathyroid storm) may lead to cardiorespiratory failure, coma and death. This is a serious risk if the patient is dehydrated. More commonly, as in this case, adenoma of one or more of the parathyroid glands results in an insidious increase in calcium levels and symptoms over many years.

Disorders of hypercalcaemia

The physiological response to hypercalcaemia is shown in Figure 10.8. In general, any excess calcium in blood is simply excreted in the urine and hypercalcaemia is relatively uncommon. There are two major pathological causes of high serum calcium levels. Oversecretion of PTH, as in the clinical case, may result from a parathyroid adenoma and is termed primary hyperparathyroidism. The second major cause of hypercalcaemia is cancer related. Various cancers produce a peptide, called parathyroid hormone-related peptide (PTHrp), which has very similar actions to PTH and causes 'hypercalcaemia of malignancy' and suppression of PTH secretion. There may also be hypercalcaemia as a result of metastases in bone causing an increased rate of bone breakdown. Rarely, very high levels of calcium-carrying proteins in the circulation may result in a falsely increased total serum calcium level, when the free or ionized calcium concentration is normal.

Interesting fact

A useful way of remembering the symptoms of hypercalcaemia:

- Stones
- Moans (depression) and
- Groans (abdominal pains)

Treatment

The treatment of primary hyperparathyroidism is initially to give fluids to restore the circulating volume and make up for losses of urine. Definitive treatment

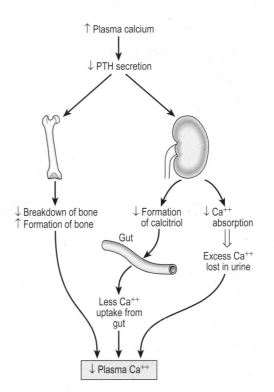

Fig. 10.8
Physiological response to hypercalcaemia. All of the mechanisms designed to conserve calcium are switched off, and the excess calcium is excreted in the urine.

is parathyroidectomy to remove a usually benign tumour of one of the four parathyroid glands. The affected gland is identified using either ultrasonography or sestamibi imaging (Fig. 10.9).

Disorders of hypocalcaemia

The physiological response to hypocalcaemia is shown in Figure 10.10. This regulatory system is totally dependent on an adequate supply of dietary calcium. If there is a chronic lack of adequate calcium uptake from the diet, then the body sacrifices bone in order to maintain plasma calcium concentrations within the normal range. For this reason it is usually possible to maintain serum calcium within the normal concentration range, however severe the dietary calcium deficiency may be.

Vitamin D deficiency

The most common reason for lack of effective calcium uptake in the gut is vitamin D deficiency. This results

HORMONAL REGULATION OF PLASMA CALCIUM AND CALCIUM METABOLISM

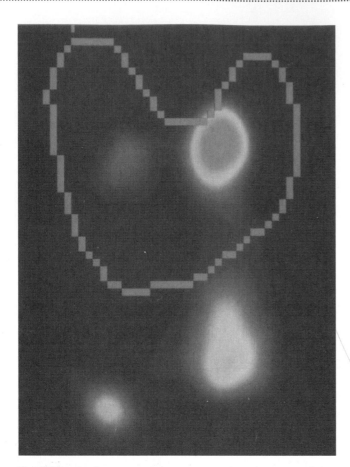

Fig. 10.9
Sestamibi scan of the parathyroid glands. The position of all four parathyroid glands is shown by scanning after uptake of radiolabelled sestamibi. Note that the left upper parathyroid gland is particularly enlarged in this patient suffering from multiple endocrine neoplasia. The outline of the thyroid gland is shown.

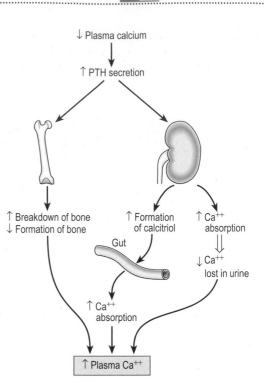

Fig. 10.10
Physiological response to hypocalcaemia. The emphasis is on maintaining plasma calcium concentrations even if this results in loss of bone mass. The only way to increase total body calcium levels is through increased uptake of dietary calcium.

from a combination of a diet lacking meat, fish and dairy products, and a lack of exposure to sunlight. It may also be seen in chronic renal failure, as the damaged kidney is no longer able to effectively perform 1-hydroxylation to produce 1,25-hydroxyvitamin D.

The bone-sacrificing effect is seen in cases of vitamin D deficiency in adults, which results in osteomalacia. Osteomalacia occurs when there is insufficient calcium (or phosphate) to mineralize newly formed bone. So a loss of bone mineral density is seen, with a greatly increased risk of fracture. In children, who are still in the phase of bone growth, vitamin D deficiency results in insufficient calcium being available both to maintain serum levels and for normal bone growth. This results in a failure of bone mineralization, leading to deformation of bones, particularly the long bones, in a condition called rickets. Although rickets is now uncommon,

it used to be a major feature of large industrial cities where poor diet, combined with lack of exposure to sunlight, resulted in many children having vitamin D deficiency.

In vitamin D deficiency, the compensation by increased secretion of PTH can make it possible for the body to maintain serum calcium levels within the normal range, and in chronic cases this can lead to a secondary hyperparathyroidism.

Parathyroid hormone deficiency

In the case of PTH deficiency, normal plasma calcium levels cannot be achieved. Hypoparathyroidism is uncommon, but causes serious and life-threatening hypocalcaemia. Without PTH it is not possible to maintain normal plasma calcium levels. Surgical removal of the parathyroid glands causes symptoms of hypocalcaemia to appear within 48 hours. The consequences of hypocalcaemia include hyperexcitability of the neuromuscular junction, which causes paraesthesia (pins and needles), tetanic contractions of skeletal muscle and even convulsions. When the respiratory muscles are affected this causes death. This hypocalcaemic *tetany* is not to be confused with *tetanus* caused by toxins produced by the bacterium *Clostridium tetani*.

Diseases of bone: osteoporosis and Paget's disease

Osteoporosis and Paget's disease are both diseases of older age that result in marked increases in bone fractures in older people. Osteoporosis is defined by the World Health Organization as 'a disease characterized by low bone mass and micro-architectural deterioration of bone tissue, leading to enhanced bone fragility and a consequent increase in fracture risk'. It is a disorder that affects 1 in 12 men but 1 in 3 women. There are two reasons why women are more susceptible to osteoporosis than men: first, women have a lower peak bone mass than men, and second, they have an accelerated rate of bone loss after the menopause. Hormone replacement therapy (HRT) used to be considered a preventive treatment for osteoporosis, but the side effects of long-term HRT use mean that it is now considered unsuitable. Lifestyle is considered to be an important factor in preventing osteoporosis, with a diet rich in vitamin D and calcium recommended together with exercise to help maintain healthy bones. In cases where osteoporosis is diagnosed, bisphosphonates are used to treat the disorder. These drugs act by suppressing osteoclast activity. They do this in two ways: by directly inhibiting recruitment of new osteoclasts and by stimulating osteoblasts to produce an osteoclast inhibitor.

Paget's disease is a poorly understood condition characterized by a marked increase in turnover in certain bones within the skeleton, while other bones remain unaffected. Paget's disease may affect only one bone or several (Fig. 10.11). It is a disease of osteoclasts, which are abnormally large and cause an increase in bone resorption. This triggers osteoblasts, which are normal, to form new bone. However, the new bone is structurally disorganized resulting in pain and increased fracture risk. It is thought to affect about 2% of the population aged over 55 years, but often occurs without symptoms. Treatment is usually with bisphosphonates.

A brief mention of calcitonin

Calcitonin is usually included in endocrine textbooks as the third hormone involved in the regulation of plasma calcium. It is a peptide hormone of 32 amino acids, secreted by the parafollicular cells of the thyroid gland

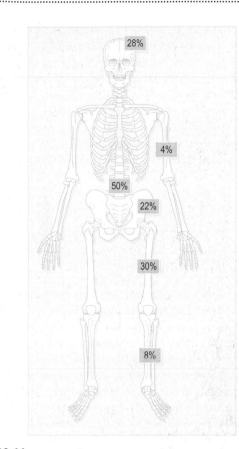

Fig. 10.11
Diagram showing the parts of the skeleton most likely to be affected by Paget's disease. (Reproduced from Chew S L, Leslie D 2006 Clinical endocrinology and diabetes: an illustrated colour text. Churchill Livingstone, Edinburgh.)

and is considered to be a calcium-lowering hormone. Its physiological role is doubtful, however, because of the total lack of pathology resulting from either hyper- or hypo-secretion of calcitonin. It has been suggested that this peptide may have a role in pregnancy to preserve the maternal skeleton, but otherwise its actions appear to be confined to lower vertebrates.

Interesting fact

Although calcitonin does not appear to be physiologically important in humans, it does have a therapeutic use. Subcutaneous injection of salmon calcitonin was the first widely used treatment for Paget's disease. It was found to halve bone turnover and improve symptoms. Its use today is limited mostly to patients who cannot tolerate bisphosphonates.

Regulation of serum phosphate

Phosphate is not as tightly regulated as serum calcium. However, there is a degree of co-regulation of calcium and phosphate. Vitamin D stimulates the uptake of both calcium and phosphate in the gut and kidney. The actions of both vitamin D and PTH on bone also cause an increase in serum phosphate levels. However, there is clear divergent regulation of calcium and phosphate in the kidney in response to PTH, which stimulates reabsorption of calcium but excretion of phosphate. This is because the likelihood of calcium phosphate crystals forming is dependent on the product of calcium concentration and phosphate concentration. If phosphate concentrations increase then calcium phosphate stones are more likely to occur in the kidney. Therefore the actions of PTH tend to keep this product fairly constant.

Self-assessment case study

Muscle pain and thin bone

Mrs Begum was a 57-year-old woman who had had pain in her back, arms and legs for several years. The pain was worse on walking or exertion. She was constantly tired. There was no history of joint swelling, stiffness or fever. She had menopause at the age of 48 years. She lived in the East End of London, UK, and had emigrated from Bangladesh about 15 years previously. Mrs Begum was a vegetarian and she always wore full hijab (traditional Muslim women's clothing) when she left the house. The clinical examination showed her to be a well looking patient. Two months previously her doctor had requested a bone mineral density scan, which showed severe osteoporosis.

Blood tests revealed:

Serum calcium	2.02 mmol/L (normal 2.20–2.60 mmol/L)
Serum phosphate	0.65 mmol/L (normal 0.8–1.2 mmol/L)
Serum creatinine	40 μmol/L (normal <120 μmol/L)
Serum PTH	12 pmol/L (normal 1.2–6.8 pmol/L)
Serum 25-hydroxyvitamin D	<13 nmol/L (normal >30 nmol/L)

Questions:

① What is the diagnosis?

② What is the mechanism of the low bone density?

③ What is the mechanism of the low phosphate concentration?

④ How may social and environmental factors have contributed to the problem?

⑤ What is the best management strategy?

Answers see page 149

Extended Matching Questions

A   Calcitonin
B   Calcitriol
C   Calcium carbonate
D   Calmodulin
E   Cholecalciferol
F   Cholesterol
G   Collagen
H   7-Dehydrocholesterol
I   Ergocalciferol
J   Hydroxyapatite
K   1-Hydroxycholecalciferol
L   25-Hydroxycholecalciferol

For each of the descriptions below, select the correct substance from the list above:

① This substance is the most important regulator of calcium absorption from the gut.

② This precursor of active vitamin D is added to margarine as a food supplement.

③ This substance can be converted to vitamin D3 by the action of sunlight.

④ This substance needs only to be hydroxylated in the kidney to become fully active vitamin D3.

⑤ This substance accounts for most of the body's calcium store.

⑥ This substance can be extracted from salmon and has been used as a treatment for Paget's disease.

Answers see page 153

MISCELLANEOUS HORMONES

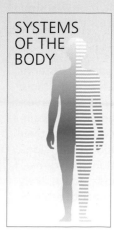

SYSTEMS
OF THE
BODY

Chapter objectives

After reading this chapter you should be able to:

① Understand the role of erythropoietin in preventing anaemia.

② Understand the role of the pineal gland and melatonin.

③ Appreciate the interactions between paracrine factors and hormones that control blood pressure.

④ Appreciate the complexity of interaction between the immune and endocrine systems, including the nature and roles of cytokines.

⑤ Appreciate the hormonal changes that occur with ageing.

⑥ Describe the principal endocrine components in the regulation of appetite.

The previous chapters of this book have dealt with the major endocrine systems of the body and their associated disorders. There are several other hormones that have not been covered and some processes that are controlled by an interaction between different systems. This chapter aims to cover the odds and ends of endocrinology and to consider some integrated systems, such as the regulation of blood pressure and volume, and the hormonal regulation of appetite.

Erythropoietin

We shall start by looking at a hormone produced by the kidney. We have already seen that the kidney is a target tissue for arginine vasopressin (AVP), aldosterone and parathyroid hormone (PTH), and that it controls the activation of vitamin D. However, the kidney is also an endocrine gland, producing a peptide hormone called erythropoietin (EPO or epo, pronounced E.P.O. and eepo respectively).

Progressive anaemia box 1

Case history

Mr Singh, a 55-year-old man with a long history of progressive chronic renal failure, is seen in outpatients for routine review. The cause of his kidney disease is chronic glomerulonephritis and the disease process can only be slowed down by good control of blood pressure. His serum creatinine level has risen from 210 μmol/L 2 years ago (estimated glomerular filtration rate [GFR] 33 mL/min) to 268 μmol/L 1 year ago (estimated GFR 28 mL/min) to 303 μmol/L at present (estimated GFR 24 mL/min).

His haemoglobin (Hb) level has fallen during recent months:

12 months ago	Hb 12.0 g/dL
6 months ago	Hb 11.4 g/dL
Today	Hb 10.6 g/dL

Other results:

Ferritin	243 ng/mL (normal)
B12 and folate	Normal
White cell and platelet counts	Normal

What is the most likely cause of Mr Singh's anaemia? How would you treat it?

Erythropoietin is a glycosylated peptide hormone secreted by the fibroblasts adjacent to the renal tubules.

It is secreted in response to either hypoxia or anaemia, but secretion is impaired in renal failure.

The major action of erythropoietin is on the bone marrow, where it stimulates the formation of red blood cells by preventing apoptosis of erthyrocyte precursor cells. An erythropoietin deficiency results in fewer red cells that contain normal amounts of iron and are a normal shape and size – in other words, a normochromic, normocytic anaemia.

Increasingly, treatment for renal failure includes replacement therapy with recombinant erythropoietin. This is indicated when other causes of anaemia, such as iron, B12 or folate deficiency, have been ruled out.

Progressive anaemia box 2

Case note: Treatment

Mr Singh's anaemia is likely to be caused by erythropoietin deficiency as a direct consequence of his renal failure. The test results indicate that it is not due to iron, B12 or folate deficiency.

He will be started on treatment with one of the forms of erythropoietin currently available. Treatment begins with a low dose and is varied over several weeks until the target Hb concentration of around 11–13 g/dl is reached. Erythropoietin is a peptide hormone, so must be given by injection. The different forms of erythropoietin have different durations of action, but treatment is typically given one to three times per week. It is also important to ensure that Mr Singh has adequate iron stores or the erythropoietin will not be as effective.

Interesting fact

It has been recognized for many years that athletes can boost their red blood cell count by training at high altitudes, where the oxygen pressure is lower, causing erythropoietin stimulation. With a higher concentration of red blood cells, athletes participating in endurance sports, such as long-distance running or cycling, will be at an advantage. More recently, with the development of recombinant erythropoietin, some athletes bypassed the altitude training and simply injected erythropoietin to boost their red blood cells. In several cases this led to pathological levels of red blood cell production (polycythaemia), resulting in stroke and thrombosis. This is likely to explain the sudden deaths of a number of athletes over recent years.

Immune–endocrine interactions: cytokines and eicosanoids

Previous chapters in this book have briefly mentioned some interactions between the immune and endocrine systems, including the effects of glucocorticoids on inflammatory and immune processes and the effects of autoimmune disease on the thyroid and pancreas. These are examples of the more obvious manifestations of the significant and complex interactions between the immune and endocrine systems. In order to look more closely at this we need to consider some of the molecules involved.

Cytokines

Cells of the immune system produce a range of chemical messengers called cytokines. However, it is not just immune cells that secrete cytokines: they are also made in vascular endothelial cells, the liver, adipocytes and many other tissues. The cytokines are families of peptides that include interleukins, erythropoietin, interferons, bone morphogenetic proteins (BMPs) and several families of growth factors, including insulin-like growth factor-1 (IGF-1), which mediates many of the effects of growth hormone, as we saw in Chapter 3. More than 100 cytokines have been identified to date.

These cytokines can act in an endocrine, paracrine or autocrine manner to bring about their effects, mediated by specific receptors, mostly of the single-transmembrane domain class, which act by activation of the Janus kinase (JAK)-STAT pathway (see Chapter 1). The different cytokines have a wide range of effects on the immune system, stimulating activation of lymphocytes and macrophages and promoting differentiation of B cells and eosinophils. Although cytokines were originally identified as messengers within the immune system, they have a somewhat broader range of effects than this, particularly in fetal development and cellular differentiation.

Cytokines also have a role in the regulation of endocrine systems. They have been implicated in the acute regulation of hormone secretion, including the release of hypothalamic stimulating factors, particularly in the response to exercise and stress. Cytokines are also known to regulate the expression of steroid-metabolizing enzymes and to have a major role in ovarian follicle maturation. They also have a longer-term role in the growth and differentiation of every endocrine tissue. It is becoming increasingly clear that cytokines are ubiquitous signalling molecules and have effects on every tissue in the body, including the endocrine system. Clinically the possibility of exploiting cytokines therapeutically is very exciting, and they are already used in the treatment of some cancers. We do not yet know how the actions of cytokines may be used in the management of endocrine disorders, and much research will be required to advance this field, but there is clearly a great deal of potential in the clinical application of cytokine research.

Eicosanoids

Some cytokines, such as interleukin-1, have a role in the promotion of inflammation. In this role they interact with a family of signalling molecules termed eicosanoids. The eicosanoids include prostaglandins, prostacyclins, thromboxanes and leukotrienes, which are all synthesized from membrane phospholipids via arachidonic acid (Fig. 11.1). Prostaglandins were

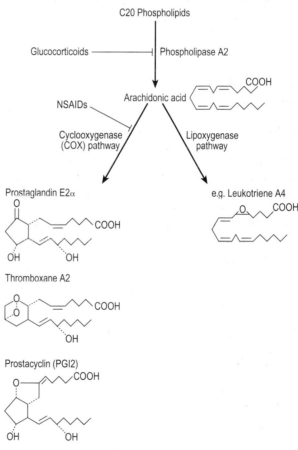

Fig. 11.1
The eicosanoids are synthesized from phospholipids in the cell membrane via the production of arachidonic acid. The action of phospholipase A2 on lipids such as linoleic acid releases arachidonic acid. The arachidonic acid is metabolized by groups of enzymes called cyclooxygenases or lipoxygenases to release prostaglandins, thromboxanes and leukotrienes. The structures of some of these compounds are shown.

given this name because they were first isolated from semen and found to be secreted by the prostate gland. It is now known that eicosanoid synthesis takes place in virtually all tissues of the body. It is known that the eicosanoids produced by the actions of one of the cyclo-oxygenase enzymes, COX2, are those most involved in pain and inflammation, so a range of drugs has been developed to specifically inhibit COX2.

In addition to their well recognized role as inflammatory mediators, the eicosanoids have several other functions, including a role in endocrine regulation, principally in the female reproductive system. In the ovary there is a rise in prostaglandin synthesis in the pre-ovulatory follicle, with the pre-ovulatory burst of luteinizing hormone increasing COX2 expression and so stimulating the release of prostaglandins E2 and F2α from follicular granulosa cells. This increase in COX2 expression and prostaglandin synthesis is now known to be an essential step in ovulation, and it has been shown that rupture of the follicle and release of the oocyte can be prevented by non-steroidal anti-inflammatory drugs (NSAIDs), which inhibit cyclo-oxygenase enzymes (see Fig. 11.1). In the light of this knowledge, women who are attempting to become pregnant are advised to avoid taking both non-selective NSAIDs and the selective COX2 inhibitors. Prostaglandins are also thought to have a role in fertilization and implantation of the embryo. In addition, prostaglandins are important in parturition as they cause ripening and dilatation of the cervix. When labour is induced, prostaglandin pessaries are used as part of the treatment.

In seminal fluid, the high concentrations of prostaglandins are thought to have an immunosuppressive effect on the female reproductive tract, allowing the sperm to reach the uterus without triggering an immune response. It has been suggested that blocking prostaglandin production by use of NSAIDs has an adverse effect on sperm quality. It has also been suggested that the age-related decline in testosterone production by Leydig cells may be related to the increased expression of COX enzymes in the testes with increasing age.

Prostacyclin and thromboxane both have a significant role in the local regulation of vascular tone, with prostacyclin acting as a vasodilator whereas thromboxane vasoconstricts (see below). They also have opposing actions on platelet aggregation, with thromboxane promoting platelet aggregation and clot formation, while prostacyclin inhibits this process.

Age-related changes in hormone secretion

It is well known that women go through the menopause at around the age of 50 years and may experience adverse effects of the associated decrease in oestrogen secretion, but the age-related decrease in other hormones is much less recognized. Men do not go through any process comparable to menopause, but there is an age-related decline in testosterone secretion, and some men experience hypogonadal symptoms associated with this. Perhaps predictably this has been termed *andropause*. The growth hormone (GH)–IGF axis also shows a marked decrease with age, a phenomenon termed *somatopause*, and, to complete the set, the adrenocortical secretion of its major androgen, dehydroepiandrosterone (DHEA), also declines with age – termed *adrenopause*.

It is not clear why age-related changes to these specific endocrine systems occur. There are no comparable patterns of change in thyroid function, for example, and the adrenopause does not include significant decreases in cortisol or aldosterone secretion.

It has been suggested that the mechanisms of andropause and somatopause might be linked, with an intact GH–IGF axis required for appropriate testicular function and an appropriate level of testosterone required to support GH secretion, but there is little evidence to support this suggestion.

Hormone replacement therapy in ageing

There are plenty of websites offering to sell you anti-ageing hormone treatments. DHEA, testosterone and GH are all readily available. But is there any evidence that they will keep you fit and healthy in old age? For most treatments the answer is 'no'. Unless somebody has a properly diagnosed hormone deficiency then there is no benefit at all in taking 'replacement therapy'. Hormone replacement therapy for post-menopausal women is well established, and testosterone replacement therapy for men with hypogonadism of old age is also a routine part of clinical practice. Administration of GH to older people who do not have a defined GH deficiency is associated with a number of adverse effects, including carpal tunnel syndrome. Probably the most popular and potentially least harmful hormonal anti-ageing treatment is DHEA. In the USA, DHEA is available over the counter and appears to be taken by a large number of individuals in a huge uncontrolled and unsupervised experiment. Although there appear to be very few side effects from taking DHEA, other than greasy skin and acne, it does not appear to have any major beneficial effects either.

Melatonin

Melatonin is a hormone involved in regulating circadian rhythms. It is produced by the pineal gland – a

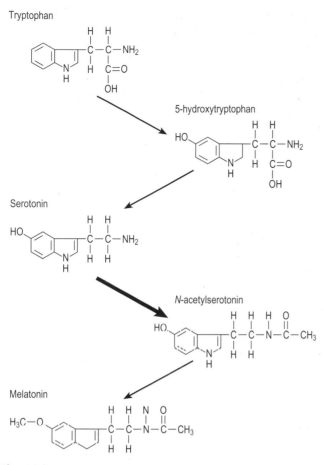

Tryptophan

5-hydroxytryptophan

Serotonin

N-acetylserotonin

Melatonin

Fig. 11.2
Synthesis of melatonin. The rate-limiting step is the conversion of serotonin to n-acetylserotonin, shown by the heavy arrow.

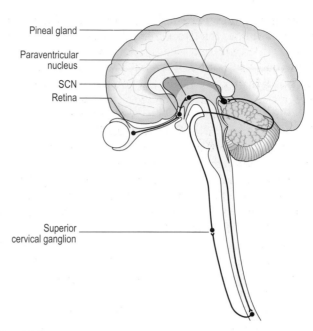

Pineal gland
Paraventricular nucleus
SCN
Retina
Superior cervical ganglion

Fig. 11.3
Pathways of pineal innervation. The signal from the retina is relayed through the suprachiasmatic nucleus (SCN) and the paraventricular nucleus, down the spinal column, returning via the superior cervical ganglion to supply the pineal gland. (Reproduced with permission from Wehr T A, Duncan W C Jr, Sher L et al 2001 A circadian signal of change of season in patients with seasonal affective disorder. Arch Gen Psychiatry 58: 1108–1114.)

small gland in the brain, named because it is the size and shape of a pine nut. Melatonin was discovered by Lerner in 1958 when he was looking for the hormone that controls melanin production in lizards. Melatonin is synthesized from tryptophan (Fig. 11.2) and its production is negatively controlled by light, so that light falling on the retina inhibits melatonin secretion. There is not a direct neural pathway from the retina to the pineal gland, but a rather complex reflex involving the cervical ganglion (Fig. 11.3). As a consequence, damage to the spinal column in this area can severely disrupt diurnal rhythms.

In humans there is a circadian rhythm of melatonin secretion, with levels being very low during the daylight hours and increasing from dusk until a peak is reached at around 3 am. Subsequently melatonin levels decline until daytime. This secretory pattern is controlled by a number of *zeitgebers* (time-givers), which include light, posture, social cues and melatonin itself. There is also a marked age dependency of melatonin secretion, with maximal secretion seen in early childhood, at around 3 years, and a gradual diminution of the amplitude of the nocturnal increase in melatonin secretion with advancing years.

The major role of melatonin is in regulating circadian rhythms of the body, including body temperature and the secretion of other hormones. It has been described as the 'circadian glue', responsible for holding the other biological rhythms in phase. In other animals, melatonin has a key role in regulating seasonal fertility by controlling the hypothalamo–pituitary–gonadal axis. There is some evidence that melatonin can affect luteinizing hormone and follicle stimulating hormone production in the human, and it has even been suggested that it may play a role in the timing of menarche, but the extent of its role remains unclear. There has been a lot of recent interest in both the antioxidant properties of melatonin and its complex interactions with the immune system. Although these functions are poorly understood, melatonin's potential as an immune modulator and in cancer treatment is being researched extensively.

Clinically melatonin has been used in the treatment of sleep disorders in older people and in regulating the body clock of 'blind-free runners', a group of profoundly blind people whose body clock does not naturally follow the usual 24-hour cycle.

Interesting fact

In the USA melatonin, like DHEA, is classified as a foodstuff and so is freely available and marketed for its supposed health benefits, one of which is the treatment of jetlag. Given at an appropriate time, melatonin may be used to phase-advance or phase-delay the circadian clock (Fig. 11.4), as desired. However, both the dose and the timing of melatonin are critical for it to have an effect.

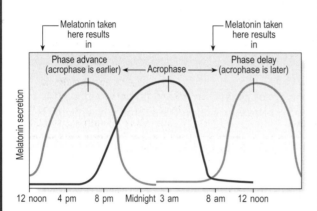

Fig. 11.4
Use of melatonin to phase shift diurnal rhythms. Melatonin secretion is stimulated by nightfall, and reaches a maximum at about 3 am. When travelling through time zones, melatonin administration can be used to phase-advance or phase-delay this secretion pattern, so resetting the biological clock for a different time zone.

Gut hormones

The first hormone to be discovered, in 1905, was a gut hormone, secretin. Over the past 100 years the study of endocrinology has flourished as we have characterized more hormones, and recognized their effects. That secretin was the first hormone to be discovered is somewhat paradoxical, as it is among the least important of all the hormones recognized today. Indeed, secretin is frequently relegated to a historical footnote in endocrine texts. Although secretin is recognized as an important gut hormone, regulating bicarbonate secretion from the pancreas, there is little pathology associated with this peptide, so it does not excite much interest. We now know that secretin is just one of a large number of polypeptide hormones secreted

by cells of the gastrointestinal tract. These hormones, their major sites of production and their main physiological actions are summarized in Table 11.1. These hormones, and the cells that produce them, are considered to be part of the 'diffuse endocrine system'. This term describes the myriad hormones secreted by endocrine and neuroendocrine cells that are scattered throughout the body, rather than being assembled into discrete endocrine glands.

Endocrine disorders involving these gastrointestinal hormones are relatively uncommon. Occasionally tumours of the gastrointestinal cells secreting these hormones are detected, but they are uncommon. The tumour most frequently seen is gastrin secreting, termed a gastrinoma, and causes Zollinger–Ellison syndrome. When a gastrinoma is detected, the patient is investigated for multiple endocrine neoplasia (MEN), a condition that is commonly found in patients presenting with gastrinoma.

Other tumours include glucagonoma, somatostatinoma and VIPoma. The latter is interesting because it presents with high volumes of watery diarrhoea, sometimes exceeding 5 litres per day. Surgical removal of the tumour is the usual treatment, although the synthetic somatostatin analogue, octreotide, may be used to treat excess vasoactive intestinal peptide (VIP) or gastrin secretion.

Multiple endocrine neoplasia (MEN)

MEN is an inherited condition that affects approximately 1 in 10 000 of the population. There are two main distinct forms of MEN, with different characteristics: MEN1 is also known as Wermer's syndrome and includes hyperparathyroidism in nearly all cases. In this condition there are often tumours of the gastrointestinal tract or pancreas, most commonly secreting gastrin or insulin. MEN2, in contrast, nearly always features medullary carcinoma of the thyroid, with phaeochromocytoma seen in around half of the patients.

As the MENs are inherited in an autosomal dominant manner, first-degree relatives of individuals with MEN may undergo genetic screening, with regular medical screening offered to those found to be carrying a *MEN* gene.

The hormonal control of appetite: fat as an endocrine tissue

Recently, with the increase in the incidence of obesity and the metabolic syndrome in the general population, there has been a huge interest in the possibility of using hormones to manipulate appetite pharmacologically.

Table 11.1
Gastrointestinal hormones

Name	Structure (no. of amino acids)	Main sites of production	Major actions
Secretin family			
Secretin	27	S cells in duodenum and jejunum	↑ Bicarbonate secretion from pancreas
Glucagon	29	A cells in upper GI tract	↑ Plasma glucose
VIP	28	Nerves throughout GI tract	↑ Intestinal secretion of electrolytes and water into lumen of gut, relaxation of sphincters
Gastrin family			
CCK	39 (+ variously sized fragments)	I cells in duodenum	↑ Pancreatic enzyme secretion; ↑ contraction of gallbladder
Gastrin	34	G cells in antral portion of gastric mucosa	↑ Gastric acid and pepsin secretion
GIP	43	K cells in duodenum and jejunum	↑ Insulin secretion
Other hormones			
GRP	27	Vagal nerve endings on G cells	↑ Gastrin secretion
Motilin	22	Enterochromaffin cells and motilin-immunopositive cells in stomach, small intestine and colon	↑ Contraction of smooth muscle and promotes GI motility
Substance P	11	Neurons throughout GI tract	↑ Motility of small intestine
Guanylin	15	Cells of intestinal mucosa	↑ Cl⁻ secretion into gut lumen
Ghrelin	28	Stomach	Stimulates appetite
Neurotensin	13	Neurons in ileum	Inhibits GI motility; ↑ ileal blood flow
Somatostatin	14	D cells in gastrointestinal mucosa	↓ Secretion of gastrin, VIP and GIP

CCK, cholecystokinin; GI, gastrointestinal; GIP, gastric inhibitory peptide; GRP, gastrin releasing peptide; VIP, vasoactive intestinal polypeptide.

It was hoped that an appetite-suppressant drug could be developed that would make dieting easier. As a result of all the research effort, we now have an improved understanding of the hormonal signals that make us hungry and also tell us when we have eaten enough. The hormonal signals regulating appetite are summarized in Figure 11.5. There are hormones produced by the gut, the pancreas and by adipose tissue that tell the appetite centre in the brain that we don't need to eat. Perhaps the most interesting of these hormones is leptin, a peptide hormone produced by fat cells.

In previous chapters we have seen that adipose tissue (fat) has a role in the conversion of testosterone to oestradiol by the action of the enzyme aromatase, which is expressed in adipose tissue. Adipocytes also secrete peptide hormones, including a range of cytokines, and leptin, a peptide hormone involved in appetite regulation. The circulating concentration of leptin is directly proportional to the absolute mass of fat in the body. Synthesis of leptin is regulated by food intake and rises after a meal. On the other hand, leptin levels decrease with fasting and it is this decrease that signals hunger. Several cases of people with a leptin deficiency have been described. These individuals have a raging hunger that is never satisfied, except by injection of leptin. In theory, it should be possible to suppress appetite by administering leptin, but in practice this doesn't work. In obese individuals there

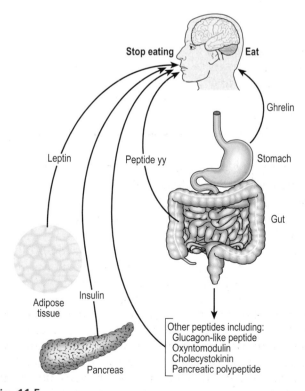

Fig. 11.5
Hormonal regulation of appetite.

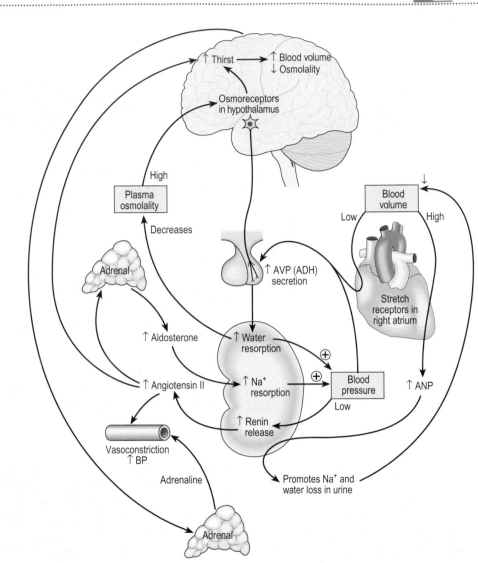

Fig. 11.6

Hormonal regulation of blood pressure, volume and osmolality. There is a complex interaction between different organs in the body to control blood volume, pressure and osmolality, which are clearly closely related. The major hormones involved are arginine vasopressin (AVP), atrial natriuretic peptide (ANP) and aldosterone. AVP, also known as anti-diuretic hormone (ADH), is secreted from the posterior pituitary and increases water resorption from urine. ANP is a hormone secreted by the right cardiac atrium that acts on the kidney to promote diuresis, with the loss of both water and sodium. Aldosterone is a mineralocorticoid secreted by the adrenal gland that increases sodium resorption in the kidney. Adrenaline and angiotensin II maintain blood pressure by acting directly on the blood vessels to produce constriction. BP, blood pressure.

is already a high level of circulating leptin and injections of more leptin has little effect on appetite.

There have been recent clinical trials on peptide YY that have had promising results. People who had infusions of this peptide ate less than people infused with saline. The problem is that the peptide has to be injected, which is not very practical, and although it reduces the amount eaten at the next meal we do not know whether it will work over a longer period of time.

In endocrinology, having several hormones doing the same job tells you that the job is important, and

we can certainly see that with appetite regulation. There is so much redundancy in this system that it's not surprising that we haven't found a magic diet pill.

Regulation of blood pressure and volume

The regulation of blood pressure and volume is achieved through the integration of many different hormonal and paracrine signals. Some of these mechanisms are shown in Figure 11.6. The actions of

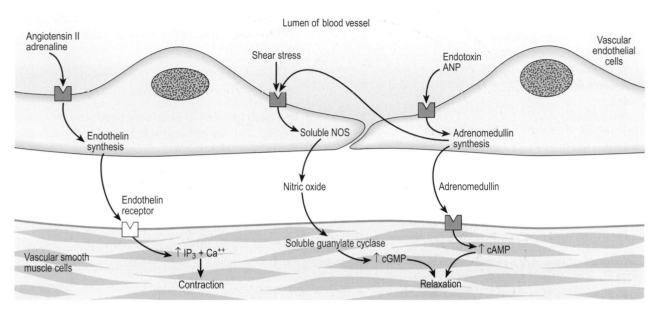

Fig. 11.7
Paracrine regulation of local vascular tone. Vascular endothelial cells secrete a range of mediators in response to hormonal and other stimuli. These mediators include nitric oxide, endothelin and adrenomedullin. ANP, atrial natriuretic peptide; cGMP/cAMP, cyclic guanosine/adenosine monophosphate; IP$_3$, inositol triphosphate; NOS, nitric oxide synthase.

aldosterone, angiotensin II and adrenaline are covered in detail in Chapter 4, and arginine vasopressin is considered in Chapter 2. The other hormone involved is atrial natriuretic peptide (ANP), a hormone secreted by the cells of the heart. This peptide acts on the kidney, via single-transmembrane ANP receptors, coupled to cyclic guanosine monophosphate (cGMP) signalling, to promote water and sodium loss in the urine. Figure 11.6 shows a simplified scheme of the major mechanisms involved in the systemic regulation of blood pressure.

In addition to the systemic regulation of blood pressure, there are several other factors that act at a local level to maintain local vascular tone (Fig. 11.7). There is evidence that nitric oxide secretion may be impaired in some patients with endocrine hypertension. It has been suggested that adrenomedullin has a role in the vasodilatation associated with septic shock.

The next 100 years of endocrinology

We started this book by observing that endocrinology is a young scientific discipline, with 2005 being recognized as the centenary of its origin. Given the wealth of knowledge that has accumulated over the last 100 years, it is tempting to speculate what an edition of this book might contain in 2105. For the centenary edition of *The Endocrinologist*, the newsletter of The Society for Endocrinology, prominent scientists and clinicians working in the field were asked to predict the status of endocrinology in 100 years' time. One of the common themes to emerge was that our understanding of the detailed interaction between different endocrine systems would be considerably greater by 2105. This 'integrated physiology', with an understanding of complex functions such as regulation of appetite, sexuality, reproduction, ageing and even body shape, could lead to tailoring of lifestyles by hormonal 'treatments'. Taken to its extreme, this argument suggests that we may even be able to use hormones to alter social behaviour. If these speculations turn out to be only partly true, it is clear that the next 100 years of hormone research will throw up many moral and ethical questions.

Extended matching questions

A   Aldosterone
B   AVP (arginine vasopressin)
C   DHEA (dehyroepiandrosterone)
D   EPO (erythropoietin)
E   Growth hormone
F   IGF-1
G   Interleukin-1
H   Melatonin
I   Parathyroid hormone
J   Peptide YY
K   Prostacyclin
L   VIP (vasoactive intestinal polypeptide)

For each of the descriptions below, choose the substance that best matches from the list above:

① Deficiency of this glycosylated peptide produced by the kidney results in a normochromic, normocytic anaemia.

② This cytokine has a role in the inflammatory process.

③ This eicosanoid is a derivative of arachidonic acid and is widely used in the body as a signalling molecule.

④ The age-related decline in this hormone's production has been termed the 'adrenopause'.

⑤ This gastrointestinal peptide is produced by neurons throughout the gut and acts to increase water and electrolyte secretion into the gut lumen.

⑥ The production of this modified amino acid is inhibited by light falling on the retina.

Answers see page 153

EXTENDED MATCHING QUESTIONS

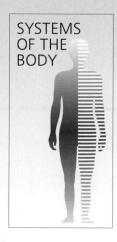

SYSTEMS
OF THE
BODY

Endocrine anatomy

A   Corpus luteum
B   Hypophyseal portal system
C   Islets of Langerhans
D   Mullerian ducts
E   Optic chiasm
F   Rathke's pouch
G   Sella turcica
H   Sphenoidal sinus
I   Suprachiasmatic nucleus
J   Vas deferens
K   Wolffian ducts
L   Zona glomerulosa

For each of the descriptions below, choose the most appropriate anatomical structure from the list above:

① This is the embryological origin of the anterior pituitary.

② The commonest surgical approach to the pituitary is via this.

③ This part of the adrenal gland is where aldosterone secreting cells are found.

④ This is the source of a thermogenic steroid hormone.

⑤ This is the embryological origin of the male reproductive system.

⑥ This is the endocrine tissue of the pancreas.

Endocrine cells I

A   Acidophil cells
B   α cells
C   Basophil cells
D   β cells
E   C cells
F   Chief cells
G   δ cells
H   G cells
I   Germ cells
J   Granulosa cells
K   Leydig cells
L   Sertoli cells

For each of the hormones below, select the cell type from the list above that produces the hormone:

① Growth hormone and prolactin.

② Activin and inhibin in the male.

③ Oestradiol.

④ Glucagon.

⑤ Parathyroid hormone.

⑥ Gastrin.

Endocrine cells II

A   Acidophil cells
B   α cells
C   Basophil cells
D   β cells
E   C cells
F   Chief cells
G   δ cells
H   G cells
I   Germ cells
J   Granulosa cells
K   Leydig cells
L   Sertoli cells

For each of the descriptions below, find the cell type from the list above that matches:

① Hormonal secretion by these cells is directly regulated by plasma calcium concentration.

② Hormonal secretion by these cells is mediated by a cell surface 'receptor' complex of GLUT2 and glucokinase.

③ Hormonal secretion by these cells is necessary for spermatogenesis, in an example of a paracrine effect.

④ Hormonal secretion by these cells is of doubtful physiological significance except possibly in pregnancy.

⑤ Hormonal secretion by these cells is inhibited by dopamine.

⑥ Hormonal secretion by these cells is not a result of *de novo* synthesis, but conversion of a precursor from adjacent cells.

Hormonal secretion

A   Active transport
B   Apocrine secretion
C   Autocrine effect
D   Ectopic secretion
E   Endocrine effect
F   Episodic secretion
G   Exocytosis
H   Facilitated diffusion
I   Neuroendocrine secretion
J   Paracrine effect
K   Phagocytosis
L   Simple diffusion

For each of the descriptions below, find the term from the list above that matches best:

① The production of ACTH by small cell carcinoma of the lung.

② The action of testosterone on Sertoli cells.

③ The action of testosterone on the brain.

④ The process of insulin release from β cells.

⑤ The process of cortisol release from zona fasciculata cells.

⑥ The process of AVP release from the posterior pituitary.

Concepts in endocrinology

A   Active transport
B   Bioassay
C   Diurnal variation
D   Dynamic test
E   Endocrine axis
F   End-product inhibition
G   Homeostatic mechanism
H   Negative feedback
I   Neuroendocrine reflex
J   Neuronal transport
K   Second messenger system
L   Synergistic action

For each of the descriptions below, find the term from the list above that best fits:

① Inhibition of GnRH by testosterone.

② Secretion of oxytocin in response to suckling.

③ The combined effect of CRH and AVP on ACTH secretion is greater than the sum of their individual effects.

④ The predictable increase and decrease in melatonin secretion over each 24-hour period.

⑤ The measurement of growth hormone in response to an oral glucose tolerance test.

⑥ Maintenance of blood sugar levels within tight limits by the opposing actions of insulin versus growth hormone, cortisol, glucagon, etc.

Named disorders

A   Addison's disease
B   Alzheimer's disease
C   Cushing's syndrome
D   Graves' disease
E   Kallman's syndrome
F   Klinefelter's syndrome
G   Kussmaul's respiration
H   Laron's syndrome
I   Paget's disease
J   Reaven's syndrome
K   Turner's syndrome
L   Zollinger–Ellison syndrome

For each of the descriptions below, pick the named disorder from the list above that best fits:

① A state of glucocorticoid excess.

② A chromosomal abnormality resulting in female phenotype, short stature and infertility.

③ A chromosomal abnormality resulting in male phenotype with impaired testicular function and infertility.

④ A feature of diabetic ketoacidosis.

⑤ A disorder caused by a gastrin-secreting tumour.

⑥ A rare cause of dwarfism due to a mutation in the code for the growth hormone receptor.

Drugs and hormones I: therapeutic uses

A   ACE inhibitor
B   Bisphosphonate
C   Bromocriptine
D   Calcitriol
E   Carbimazole
F   Desmopressin
G   Glucocorticoid
H   Iodine
I   Metformin
J   Mifepristone
K   Statin
L   Sulphonylurea

For each of the descriptions below, choose the name from the list above that best matches:

① This synthetic dopamine antagonist is used to shrink prolactinomas and control hyperprolactinaemia.

② This antithyroid drug is used to control an overactive thyroid gland.

③ This biguanide is used in the management of non-insulin-dependent diabetes mellitus.

④ This synthetic peptide is used in the management of diabetes insipidus.

⑤ This HMG CoA reductase inhibitor is used in the management of the metabolic syndrome.

⑥ This enzyme inhibitor is used in the management of hypertension.

Drugs and hormones II: adverse effects

A   Buserelin
B   Carbamazepine
C   Chlorpromazine

D   Chlorpropamide
E   Enalapril
F   Lithium
G   NSAID
H   Prednisolone
I   Progestin
J   Stanozolol
K   Sulphonylurea
L   Warfarin

For each of the descriptions below, choose the name from the list above that best matches:

① An anti-inflammatory drug that can inhibit ovulation.

② This drug causes increased renal sensitivity to AVP, resulting in oliguria.

③ A dopamine antagonist that can result in hyperprolactinaemia.

④ An anti-epileptic that can cause SIADH.

⑤ A drug of abuse that can cause male and female infertility.

⑥ A synthetic glucocorticoid whose use can be associated with mood disorders.

Drugs and hormones III: The adrenals

A   Androstenedione
B   Atenolol
C   Dehydroepiandrosterone
D   11-Deoxycortisol
E   Dexamethasone
F   Glycerrhitinic acid
G   Hydrocortisone
H   Phenoxybenzamine
I   Phosphatidylinositol
J   Prednisolone
K   Propranolol
L   Spironolactone

For each of the descriptions below, choose the name from the list above that best matches:

① This substance, found in liquorice, is an inhibitor of 11-β hydroxysteroid dehydrogenase.

② This is the name given to cortisol when it is administered as a drug.

③ This is the only synthetic glucocorticoid that does not have significant mineralocorticoid action.

④ This is an aldosterone receptor antagonist.

⑤ This α-adrenergic receptor antagonist is used to control the effects of a phaeochromocytoma before surgery.

⑥ This naturally occurring adrenal steroid is marketed as a 'medicine' on the grounds that its production declines with age, so taking it as a drug will reverse the ageing process.

Endocrine investigation

A   Chromosomal analysis
B   Cold stressor test
C   Dexamethasone suppression test
D   DEXA scan
E   FDG-PET scan
F   Heel-prick blood test
G   Insulin tolerance test
H   MIBG scan
I   MRI brain scan
J   Oral glucose tolerance test
K   Urinary hCG immunoassay
L   Water deprivation test

For each of the descriptions below, choose the test from the list above that best matches:

① Investigation of raised blood cortisol levels.

② Detection of phaeochromocytoma.

③ Dynamic test of GH and ACTH used in the investigation of hypopituitarism.

④ Detection of congenital hypothyroidism in neonates.

⑤ Investigation of male primary hypogonadism.

⑥ Detection of pregnancy.

Endocrine biochemistry

A   Low calcium level in blood
B   Low glucose level in blood
C   Low pH level in blood
D   Low potassium level in blood
E   Low sodium level in blood
F   Raised calcium level in blood
G   Raised cholesterol level in blood
H   Raised free fatty acid level in blood
I   Raised glucose level in blood
J   Raised pH level in blood
K   Raised potassium level in blood
L   Raised sodium level in blood

For each of the descriptions below, choose the biochemical finding from the list above that best matches:

① The result of ectopic PTHrp secretion by tumours.

② Stimulates renin release by the kidney.

③ Characteristic feature of mineralocorticoid excess, along with hypertension.

④ Raised levels of HbA1c correlate with this.

⑤ Feature of the metabolic syndrome managed by statins.

⑥ Kussmaul's respiration is the body's attempt to compensate for this.

Hormone deficiency

A Calcitonin
B Cortisol
C Adrenaline (epinephrine)
D Erythropoietin
E Follicle stimulating hormone
F Gastrin
G Growth hormone
H Insulin
I Luteinizing hormone
J Parathyroid hormone
K Testosterone
L Thyroxine

For each of the clinical scenarios below, choose the hormone from the list above that is most likely to be deficient:

① Hyperglycaemia, ketoacidisis, polyuria and polydipsia in a 15-year-old boy who was previously well.

② Normochromic, normocytic anaemia in a 55-year-old man with chronic renal failure.

③ Tetany in a 60-year-old woman who has just undergone total thyroidectomy.

④ Infertility and loss of secondary sex characteristics in a 34-year-old man who has recently had severe mumps orchitis.

⑤ Tiredness, lethargy, depression and cold intolerance in a 40-year-old woman who has been taking lithium for a year.

⑥ Weakness, vomiting, dehydration, hypotension and hypoglycaemia in a moribund 28-year-old woman who had recently been on a prolonged course of prednisolone for asthma.

Hormone excess

A ACTH
B Aldosterone
C AVP
D Adrenaline (epinephrine)
E GH
F Oestradiol
G Oxytocin
H Prolactin
I PTH
J Testosterone
K TSH
L VIP

For each of the clinical descriptions below, choose the hormone from the list above whose excess is most likely to be responsible for the symptoms:

① Asymptomatic (unless there are space-occupying effects).

② Impaired glucose tolerance, moon face, truncal obesity with wasting of arms and legs, and easy bruising.

③ Impaired glucose tolerance, coarsening of facial features, and increased size of hands, feet and lower jaw.

④ Impaired glucose tolerance, hypertension, tachycardia, palpitations, sweating and pupillary dilatation.

⑤ Male gynaecomastia and milk expression from breasts.

⑥ Profuse, watery diarrhoea.

And finally...

A Blackbird
B Cow
C Dog
D Gadfly
E Guinea-pig
F Hamster
G Human
H Lizard
I Rat
J Rattlesnake
K Salmon
L Toad

For each of the descriptions below, choose the most appropriate animal from the list above:

① The Greek name for this animal, literally meaning 'frenzy', gives us the word 'oestrous'.

② This domestic animal has one oestrous cycle per year.

③ This domestic animal has two oestrous cycles per year.

④ This animal was used for a successful bioassay pregnancy test for several decades.

⑤ This animal has been used as a source of calcitonin for medicinal use.

⑥ Melatonin was discovered in this animal.

ANSWERS

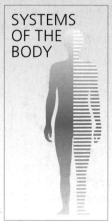

SYSTEMS
OF THE
BODY

Self-assessment case study answers

Chapter 3

① What is the diagnosis?

Microprolactinoma of the anterior pituitary. The tumour is less than 10 mm and is therefore a microadenoma.

② What is the mechanism of amenorrhoea?

The high prolactin level suppresses the production of LH and FSH and also blocks the response of the ovary to LH and FSH. This dual action leads to lack of ovulation and low oestradiol levels. The uterus is not primed by oestradiol and a lack of periods is the result.

③ What is the correct management strategy?

The best treatment is to use a dopamine agonist. Prolactin is normally under tonic inhibition by the neurotransmitter dopamine. Synthetic dopamine agonists (such as bromocriptine or cabergoline) are able to bind and powerfully stimulate the dopamine receptors on the microprolactinoma, and the tumours are usually still partially sensitive to dopamine control. This results in tumour shrinkage and normalization of the prolactin level. The treatment will not cure the patient because the tumour will regrow if it is stopped; however, the condition can be well controlled for life on these drugs. The patient should be warned that treatment will restore ovulation and therefore fertility.

Chapter 4

① What is the likeliest diagnosis for the adrenal mass?

Adrenocortical adenoma. An adenoma that is found during the course of investigations for another problem is often called an adrenal incidentaloma. In this case the main problem was gallstone colic and the adrenal mass was discovered incidentally. Although the adrenal mass was incidental, it still may cause symptoms (see answer 3 below).

② What are three alternative, but less likely, diagnoses?

Adrenocortical carcinoma, adrenomedullary phaeochromocytoma or adrenal metastasis.

③ What clinical features might suggest the mass was a functioning lesion?

Hypertension, obesity, red round face – suggesting over-secretion of cortisol causing Cushing's syndrome.

④ What tests would determine whether the mass was functioning or non-functioning?

Assessment of adrenocortical and adrenomedullary function. Adrenocortical adenomas may over-secrete glucocorticoids, androgens or mineralocorticoids. These may be tested by measuring serum levels of cortisol, plasma ACTH (for glucocorticoid over-secretion); serum DHEA/S, androstenedione and testosterone (androgens); and plasma renin and serum aldosterone (mineralocorticoid function). Adrenomedullary function is usually tested by measurement of adrenaline (epinephrine) or noradrenaline (norepinephrine), or metabolites (metnoradrenaline) in the blood and urine.

⑤ If surgical treatment is needed, what is the surgical anatomy of the adrenal blood vessels?

The adrenal artery arises directly from the abdominal aorta superior to the origin of the right renal artery, and runs behind the inferior vena cava to the right adrenal gland. The adrenal vein is a short fat vessel running directly into the inferior vena cava. The surgeon must control the short fat adrenal vein before removal of the adrenal. The main risk is severe venous bleeding because of tears in the inferior vena cava or incomplete ligation of the adrenal vein. This can be very difficult to control and may be fatal. A right adrenalectomy should be attempted only by expert surgeons.

Chapter 5

① List the anatomical structures that were compressed by the neck mass resulting in the symptoms experienced by Mrs Zabedic.

Trachea, oesophagus, thoracic inlet, internal jugular vein (possibly also the superior vena cava).

② What is the likeliest diagnosis of the neck mass?

Iodine deficiency goitre with retrosternal extension (likely haemorrhage to explain sudden deterioration of symptoms).

③ Which of the following terms best describes the thyroid function of Mrs Zabedic: euthyroid, hyperthyroid or hypothyroid?

Euthyroid.

④ List the structures that may be damaged by surgical removal of the neck mass.

Recurrent laryngeal nerve, parathyroid glands (trachea, common carotid arteries, internal jugular veins, oesophagus much less likely).

⑤ What hormonal deficiency may explain the symptoms on the second day after surgery?

Parathyroid hormone (PTH), resulting in low calcium levels, caused by removal of the parathyroid glands at the same time as the thyroid (see Chapter 10).

Chapter 6

① What is the mechanism for the raised LH and FSH?

The main mechanism is the loss of feedback suppression of LH and FSH by testosterone. Testicular damage results in lowered testosterone and inhibin levels. The pituitary and hypothalamus then synthesize and release more gonadotropins. Chemotherapy is one of the commonest causes of testicular failure. Viral infections (mumps) or trauma are other recognized causes.

② What is the diagnosis?

Chemotherapy-induced testicular failure. The toxicity of chemotherapy damages both the germ cells and Leydig cells. Sperm should have been stored before starting chemotherapy to allow future fertility treatment with artificial insemination.

③ What are the long-term risks and benefits of testosterone replacement?

The main long-term benefits are to improve symptoms such as flushing and fatigue, thereby improving quality of life. Testosterone is also required for maintenance of bone density and probably for vascular health. The disadvantages are that testosterone therapy may increase prostate size and possibly the risk of prostate carcinoma. It may cause polycythaemia in patients at risk of hypoxia (e.g. due to respiratory disease). This is because testosterone is a driver of erythropoiesis (red cell production), as is hypoxia.

Chapter 7

① How do you interpret the blood test?

The tests show hypogonadotropic hypogonadism. The gonadal sex steroids (oestradiol and testosterone) are undetectable. This is the direct cause of a lack of uterine bleeding. However, the LH and FSH levels are very low because the lack of negative feedback from oestradiol should stimulate LH and FSH secretion. This indicates that the problem is hypothalamic or pituitary, rather than primarily ovarian.

② What other investigations may be helpful?

MRI of the brain, hypothalamus and pituitary to exclude a neoplasm of the pituitary; smell test (anosmia – reduced smell – is a feature of Kallmann's syndrome, which is a rare genetic cause of hypogonadotropic hypogonadism); serum prolactin (high prolactin levels may cause hypogonadotropic hypogonadism); anterior pituitary hormones. In view of her low BMI it would also be sensible to question her more closely about her body image (does she think she is fat?) and her eating habits (does she restrict her calorie intake?).

③ What is the differential diagnosis, starting with the likeliest?

The most likely diagnosis is weight and exercise-related amenorrhoea, raising the possibility of anorexia nervosa. Other differential diagnoses include: prolactinoma; non-functioning pituitary adenoma; Kallmann's syndrome; inflammatory and infectious disease of the hypothalamus and pituitary (these are unlikely without other hormonal deficits or symptoms).

Chapter 8

① What is the diagnosis?

Turner's syndrome, a chromosomal disorder. This is a classical presentation. The other features are cardiovascular and renal anomalies, autoimmune disorders (thyroid disease and diabetes mellitus) and skeletal abnormalities.

② What is the cause of the cardiac murmur and raised blood pressure?

Coarctation of the aorta – a narrowing of the aorta, usually at the level of the ductus arteriosus. This causes blood pressure to be high in the upper limbs (branches of the subclavian artery exit the aorta before the narrowing). The arterial supply to the lower body is reduced by the narrowing. The main complications of coarctation of the aorta are stroke and myocardial infarction.

③ What test confirms the diagnosis?

A karyotype. Blood is taken fresh to the laboratory and white cells are cultured. The chromosomes are stained and examined microscopically. Fluorescent probes to genetic loci may also be used (fluorescent in-situ hybridization, FISH). The classical Turner's karyotype is 45XO. Some patients show mosaicism, where some cells are normal 46XX, whereas others are 45XO.

④ Will she have periods when treated with hormone replacement therapy?

Yes. HRT is needed to allow bone maturation and secondary sexual characteristics. She will have a uterus. Although the ovaries are usually only small streaks of tissue and contain no or few follicles (called streak gonads), the mullerian structures will persist in this patient as this is the default developmental state. Once oestradiol has been given, the endometrium will develop and menstrual bleeding will occur.

⑤ Will she be fertile?

No. She will be able to conceive only by means of IVF with donor ova. She will have no follicles of her own due to the undeveloped ovaries (streak gonads). However, it would be possible for her to carry a pregnancy to term if a donor provided an ovum and IVF was performed and the embryo implanted.

Chapter 9

① How does knowledge of endogenous insulin production help in the interpretation of her biochemical investigations?

Insulin is expressed as a single precursor polypeptide chain known as pre-pro-insulin, which must be cleaved by proteolytic enzymes – a mechanism known as post-translational processing. A connecting peptide (C-peptide) is cleaved from the A- and B-peptide, leaving the mature insulin molecule. Insulin and C-peptide flow to the liver in the portal circulation, where insulin acts and is consumed. C-peptide is extracted less efficiently by the liver and is detectable at higher levels in the general circulation. Her undetectable C-peptide levels indicate that no endogenous insulin is being made. Thus, the high serum insulin level must be derived from an exogenous source. The high insulin level is clearly inappropriate for the low glucose level.

② What is the likeliest diagnosis?

The patient has insulin-induced hypoglycaemia causing neuroglycopenia. The insulin was from an exogenous source. When questioned, the patient admitted to having had an argument with her boyfriend, who had ended their relationship 2 days earlier. She had taken the insulin supplies from a patient she had seen as a student and self-injected the insulin.

③ Her dextrose infusion is stopped at 12 hours, but her confusion returns. What is the likeliest diagnosis?

She may have taken a further injection of insulin, or, more likely, she injected herself with a long-acting insulin.

④ What is the purpose of the urine sulphonylurea test?

Sulphonylurea drugs stimulate excess endogenous insulin to cause hypoglycaemia. This was a possible diagnosis. However, the C-peptide level is high in sulphonylurea poisoning, because the insulin is endogenous.

Chapter 10

① What is the diagnosis?

Osteomalacia and severe vitamin D deficiency. There is secondary hyperparathyroidism and a myopathy and myalgia, all due to vitamin D deficiency.

② What is the mechanism of the low bone density?

The lack of vitamin D results in poor absorption of calcium from the gut. This is sensed by the calcium sensing receptor on the parathyroid glands and increased PTH is secreted. PTH causes resorption of skeletal calcium stores leading to a lack of bone mineralization and increased risk of fracture. Furthermore, the lack of vitamin D causes a loss of osteoblast function and thus defective bone mineralization.

③ What is the mechanism of the low phosphate concentration?

PTH stimulates phosphate excretion from the kidney.

④ How may social and environmental factors have contributed to the problem?

The patient lives in London, UK, which is at a high latitude. There is little sun exposure and very low skin production of vitamin D precursors, particularly in the winter months from November to April. In addition, she wore a head and face covering for religious and cultural reasons. Her diet was likely to be relatively low in vitamin D, which would compound the lack of vitamin D formation in her skin. To add further to the problem, the flour used to make chapatis contains phytates, which inhibit calcium absorption from the gut.

⑤ What is the best management strategy?

A daily oral vitamin D supplement taken for life. The treatment was monitored by serum calcium and vitamin D measurements and a repeat bone densitometry scan about 12 months after treatment.

Extended matching question answers

Chapter 1

① G (noradrenaline)

The catecholamines noradrenaline (norepinephrine), adrenaline (epinephrine) and dopamine are all modified tyrosine residues. The only other modified amino acid in the list is thyroxine, which is not a catecholamine. Tyrosine, of course, is not a hormone (as you will have spotted).

② E (growth hormone)

ANP, insulin, prolactin and TSH are also peptide hormones, but only growth hormone has the diurnal secretion described here. TSH levels, like T4, are virtually constant over 24 hours.

③ A (aldosterone)

Cortisol and testosterone are the other steroid hormones in the list, but each of these has a specific carrier protein: CBG and SHBG respectively. Aldosterone circulates in very low concentrations, mostly bound loosely to plasma albumin. Cholesterol is a steroid and is the precursor of all steroid hormones, but is not itself a hormone.

④ B (ANP)

Other single-transmembrane domain receptors such as growth factor receptor and cytokine receptors, also do not use traditional second messengers.

⑤ J (thyroxine)

Like steroid hormones, the thyroid hormones act on intracellular receptors to regulate gene transcription.

⑥ F (insulin)

As a class, growth factor receptors seem to be unique in having in-built tyrosine kinase activity, which is used in signal transduction.

Chapter 2

① G (magnocellular neurons)

AVP is synthesized in the cell bodies of the magnocellular neurons in the hypothalamus and transported down neuronal projections into the posterior pituitary, where it is released.

② C (collecting ducts of the kidney)

V_2 receptors mediate the effects of AVP on water balance. Other effects of AVP, on vascular smooth muscle and the pituitary, are mediated by V_1 receptors. V_2 receptors are also found on vascular endothelial cells, which makes this a hard question.

③ B (aortic arch)

Baroreceptors, which respond to a fall in blood pressure, are also found in the carotid artery, but that was not one of the options. The baroreceptors found in the right atrium respond to a fall in blood volume. Both types of baroreceptor can contribute to increased AVP secretion but the principal regulation of AVP is via osmolality.

④ A (anterior pituitary)

AVP acts synergistically with CRH to stimulate ACTH release from the anterior pituitary. This effect is mediated by V_{1b} receptors.

⑤ E (hypothalamus)

Hypothalamic chemoreceptors are the most important factor in the regulation of AVP secretion, due to their sensitivity to plasma osmolality.

⑥ J (posterior pituitary)

Like AVP, oxytocin is synthesized in the hypothalamus and reaches the posterior pituitary by neuronal transport. It is released into the circulation from the posterior pituitary.

Chapter 3

① D (dopamine)

Dopamine is a modified amino acid and catecholamine.

② J (somatostatin)

The sensitivity of growth hormone secretion to somatostatin inhibition is exploited therapeutically in the use of octreotide, a synthetic somatostatin analogue. Octreotide can be used to reduce the size of growth hormone-secreting adenomas before surgical removal of the tumour.

③ L (TSH)

For reasons that are not entirely clear, the order in which space-occupying tumours affect pituitary function is usually growth hormone first, then LH and FSH, with ACTH and TSH being the most resistant to damage. Can you explain why prolactin secretion may be paradoxically increased by a space-occupying tumour?

④ H (LH)

LH and FSH both have actions on the gonads so, as the name suggests, are produced by gonadotroph cells and are collectively termed the gonadotropins.

⑤ A (ACTH)

ACTH is the smallest anterior pituitary hormone and is formed by splitting of the POMC (pro-opiomelanocortin) peptide. Other products of POMC processing include β-endorphin and met-enkephalin.

⑥ F (growth hormone)

Growth hormone acts to increase plasma glucose levels through a combination of decreased peripheral uptake of glucose and increased hepatic gluconeogenesis. In acromegaly, where there is excess growth hormone production, these effects can result in impaired glucose tolerance or even outright diabetes mellitus.

⑦ G (IGF-1)
Yes, sometimes it really is this obvious.

⑧ I (prolactin)
The regulation of prolactin is unusual in that it is principally under tonic inhibitory control by dopamine. The consequence of this is that prolactin is increased by factors that reduce the amount of dopamine reaching the anterior pituitary. For example, space-occupying tumours that compress the pituitary stalk will decrease the inhibitory effect of dopamine and therefore increase prolactin secretion at a time when the levels of other pituitary hormones are decreasing.

Chapter 4

① K (pregnenolone)
The rate-limiting step of steroidogenesis is the conversion of cholesterol to pregnenolone. Strictly speaking it is the rate of delivery of cholesterol to the enzyme that catalyses this reaction that limits the rate of steroidogenesis. This is achieved by the StAR protein.

② A (aldosterone)
Other steroids, even glucocorticoids, can have some mineralocorticoid effects, but aldosterone is by far the most potent. In some forms of CAH, notably those affecting 11β-hydroxylase, the excess of 11-deoxycorticosterone and 11-deoxycortisol produces a sufficient mineralocorticoid effect so that salt wasting is not seen.

③ F (dehydroepiandrosterone)
Not only is DHEA and its sulphated form (DHEAS) the major product of the human adrenal cortex, but it also shows the most marked changes with age. Levels of DHEA rise during childhood and puberty, plateau in early adulthood, and then decline progressively throughout the rest of life.

④ J (17α-hydroxyprogesterone)
The lack of 21-hydroxylase activity blocks the conversion of 17α-hydroxyprogesterone to 11-deoxycortisol, and of progesterone to 11-deoxycorticosterone. The excess of 17α-hydroxyprogesterone leads to increased levels of androstenedione, a weak androgen.

⑤ E (cortisol)
This is just another way of asking 'Which is the major glucocorticoid?'. Cortisol also has effects on protein catabolism, the immune system and blood pressure.

⑥ C (cholesterol)
Steroid secreting cells do not store the hormone product, but instead keep large stores of the precursor, cholesterol, in lipid droplets in the cells.

Chapter 5

① I (recurrent laryngeal nerve)
The recurrent laryngeal nerve, which lies between the thyroid lobe and the trachea on each side, is particularly susceptible to damage during thyroid surgery. Unilateral section can result in hoarseness of speech.

② H (parathyroid glands)
The parathyroid glands are usually multiple, so it is uncommon to remove all of them accidentally except during total thyroidectomy. The parathyroid glands produce PTH, which is important in the regulation of blood calcium levels. Low blood calcium concentration can produce tingling in the fingers and lips, and weakness.

③ L (trachea)
The trachea appears dark on chest radiography as it is an air-filled cavity, so it can be clearly seen. Swelling of the thyroid can be so great as to push the trachea to one side; this shows up on a chest radiograph as 'tracheal deviation'.

④ D (heart)
Palpitations and tachycardia are common in thyrotoxicosis and may be alleviated by propranolol, a β-adrenergic antagonist. Other cardiac effects of thyrotoxicosis, which may not be improved by propranolol, are atrial fibrillation and heart failure.

⑤ B (eyes)
A build-up of tissue behind the eyes pushes them forwards, making them appear to bulge out. Other eye effects are lid retraction, which can be demonstrated by 'lid-lag', where the patient is asked to follow the examiner's finger moving downwards and the eyelid follows in a delayed and jerky manner.

⑥ J (skin)
Myxoedema is a thickening of the skin, particularly seen on the anterior surfaces of the lower limbs (hence pre-tibial myxoedema).

Chapter 6

① H (luteinizing hormone, LH)
This is easy to remember from L for LH and L for Leydig cells.

② A (activin)
Of the two peptide products of Sertoli cells, activin activates the axis and inhibin inhibits it.

③ **B (androgen binding protein, ABP)**
Whereas the secondary sexual characteristics are controlled by dihydrotestosterone, testosterone itself is required to maintain spermatogenesis. Because testosterone is lipid soluble and tends to diffuse across cell membranes, androgen binding protein is used to maintain high testicular concentrations.

④ **L (testosterone)**
Perhaps surprisingly, androgens and oestrogens may be interconverted by the enzyme aromatase. Some of the actions of testosterone, particularly in the brain, require prior conversion to oestradiol.

⑤ **G (inhibin)**
It is not clear why this should be, but inhibin provides a useful test of Sertoli cell function in fertility clinics.

⑥ **J (stanozolol)**
This is the only synthetic androgen in the list: androstenedione is on the metabolic pathway to testosterone and dihydrotestosterone is the peripherally active androgen formed by the action of 5α-reductase on testosterone. Stanozolol is a synthetic analogue of testosterone that is active orally and popular with, for example, body builders.

Chapter 7

① **D (menstrual cycle day 14)**
This profile is characteristic of the time around ovulation when the LH surge has stimulated oestradiol levels but the corpus luteum has not yet formed, so progesterone levels are low.

② **J (pregnancy third trimester)**
The presence of detectable hCG indicates pregnancy but the levels of hPL, progesterone and prolactin rise throughout pregnancy, so the combination of only moderately raised hCG (down from the first trimester peak) with very high levels of hPL, progesterone and prolactin indicates the third trimester.

③ **E (menstrual cycle day 21)**
Here, the absence of hCG rules out pregnancy. High progesterone levels therefore indicate a functioning corpus luteum. Oestradiol levels, which have declined from their peak, along with low LH and FSH levels, are part of this characteristic pattern. This is the classical time to test for the functional integrity of the female reproductive system by measuring levels of these hormones.

④ **G (polycystic ovarian syndrome, PCOS)**
This profile is pathognomonic for PCOS; in other words, there is no other diagnosis that could account for this

pattern. Androstenedione is a weak androgen, and this accounts for some of the masculinizing effects of this condition. Again, low progesterone concentration indicates the absence of a functional corpus luteum, particularly as the measurement would normally be taken at day 21 of the cycle (compare with the profile for 3). The high LH/FSH ratio is characteristic of PCOS.

⑤ **H (pregnancy first trimester)**
Once more, detectable hCG indicates pregnancy, and the combination of high hCG with low hPL levels suggests early pregnancy (i.e. first trimester). Although progesterone levels are high in the first trimester relative to levels during the menstrual cycle, progesterone concentration increases greatly during the third trimester.

⑥ **L (post-menopause)**
We couldn't resist this one, even though menopause is in the next chapter! The clues are undetectable hCG, which tells us that the woman is not pregnant, and very high gonadotropin levels, which are obviously having no effect on ovarian function. The answer cannot be pre-menarche (absent puberty), because the woman has had two normal pregnancies, or anorexia nervosa, because the concentration of gonadotropins would not be greatly raised.

Chapter 8

① **H (medroxyprogesterone acetate)**
This is the most commonly used long-term contraceptive. The compound is slowly hydrolysed to release a progestogen, with almost 100% contraceptive efficacy.

② **J (mifepristone; RU486)**
The simplest form of morning-after pill, which probably decreases the chance of implantation, is a high dose of combined oestrogen and progestogen. This is most effective within the first 24 hours after unprotected sex. Mifepristone is effective both as a morning-after pill and for inducing termination of pregnancy at a later stage, so is more useful if more than 24 hours have elapsed since intercourse.

③ **C (clomiphene)**
Clomiphene is an anti-oestrogen that works by blocking oestrogen receptors. This prevents oestrogen negative feedback to the pituitary, and therefore leads to the release of gonadotropins, which can induce ovulation.

④ **B (buserelin)**
Endogenous GnRH secretion from the hypothalamus is pulsatile and stimulates LH and FSH production by the pituitary. Buserelin, a GnRH agonist, provides constant stimulation, which inhibits LH and FSH secretion.

⑤ **F (genistein)**

Phyto-oestrogens are plant oestrogens or oestrogen-like compounds. They are found in a variety of plants and some foods, including soy products. They are marketed as 'natural' HRT.

⑥ **K (norethisterone)**

Norethisterone is the classic progestin or progestogen used in the oral contraceptive pill. The other commonly used progestin is levonorgestrel.

Note: Shame on you if you answered G or L to any of the questions. KY jelly can be used as a vaginal lubricant (not active orally) and silphium is the contraceptive plant of classical antiquity that became extinct centuries ago.

Chapter 9

① **K (phosphorylation cascade)**

Insulin activation of its receptor triggers a phosphorylation cascade, which starts with insulin receptor substrate (IRS) phosphorylation.

② **D (glycation [glycosylation] of haemoglobin)**

All tissues and cells have proteins that are subject to glycosylation, the extent of which depends on the prevailing concentration of glucose. Assay of glycosylated haemoglobin (HbA1c) is easy from a simple blood sample and indicates average blood glucose levels over the past couple of months.

③ **L (proteolysis)**

Pro-insulin is processed to become mature insulin by having the middle of the peptide sequence removed by proteolysis. Mature insulin is a pair of peptide chains joined by disulphide bridges; the connecting peptide, which is also released, is C-peptide.

④ **B (exocytosis)**

Mature insulin is stored in granules in β cells. Glucose entering the islet cells via the GLUT2 transporter results in a sequence of events that culminates in exocytosis of the insulin-containing granules.

⑤ **E (glycogenolysis)**

At the same time as promoting the uptake of glucose by peripheral cells, insulin also acts to prevent the further release of glucose into the blood from the liver. It achieves this by inhibiting glycogen breakdown.

⑥ **I (lipolysis)**

Although the main effects of glucagon are on the liver, it also acts on adipose tissue to stimulate lipolysis. In insulin deficiency, this action of glucagon contributes to ketoacidosis.

Chapter 10

① **B (calcitriol)**

Calcitriol, also known as active vitamin D and 1,25-dihydroxyvitamin D, acts on cells in the gastrointestinal tract to increase production of calcium transport proteins.

② **I (ergocalciferol)**

Ergocalciferol, also known as vitamin D2, is derived from yeast and fungus and is added to margarines as a supplement in order to prevent vitamin D deficiency. Calcium carbonate is added to flour.

③ **H (7-dehydrocholesterol)**

This cholesterol derivative, found in skin, can be converted to vitamin D3, which is also known as cholecalciferol. Vitamin D3 can also be obtained in the diet from dairy produce, oily fish and liver.

④ **L (25-hydroxycholecalciferol)**

Vitamins D2 and D3 need to undergo a double hydroxylation to form calcitriol. What this question is really asking is which of these hydroxylations occurs in the kidney. The answer is that 25-hydroxylation happens in the liver and 1-hydroxylation in the kidney.

⑤ **J (hydroxyapatite)**

Hydroxyapatite is a complex mineral combining calcium and phosphate that is held in a collagen matrix to form bone.

⑥ **A (calcitonin)**

Physiologically, calcitonin does not seem to be very important in the human. Like many hormones, calcitonin has a very different function in lower vertebrates. It is produced in large quantities by salmon leading to its former use as a therapy for Paget's disease.

Chapter 11

① **D (erythropoietin)**

The main action of EPO is to stimulate red blood cell formation in the bone marrow. EPO deficiency results in fewer red cells, but a normal shape and size and with normal amounts of iron.

② **G (interleukin-1)**

Interleukin-1 has a role in the promotion of inflammation and interacts with the eicosanoids, which include prostaglandins, prostacyclins, thromboxanes and leukotrienes.

③ **K (prostacyclin)**

Also known as prostaglandin I2, prostacyclin is one of the eicosanoids produced from arachidonic acid via the cyclo-oxygenase pathway.

④ **C (DHEA)**
DHEA shows a characteristic decline with age. Unlike the menopause, the so-called adrenopause is a gradual process over a long period of time.

⑤ **L (VIP)**
Interestingly, cholera toxin has its effects by directly activating the VIP signal transduction pathway and prevents it from switching off. This accounts for the massive watery diarrhoea seen in cholera infection.

⑥ **H (melatonin)**
Melatonin, produced by the pineal gland, is secreted mostly at night and has a variety of roles ranging from zeitgeber to anti-oxidant.

Chapter 12

Endocrine anatomy
① **F (Rathke's pouch)**
The anterior pituitary is ectodermal in origin and derives from Rathke's pouch, which is an outgrowth of the buccal cavity.

② **H (sphenoidal sinus)**
Pituitary tumours can be removed by a surgical approach through the nose and sphenoidal sinus.

③ **L (zona glomerulosa)**
The other two parts of the adrenal cortex are the zona fasciculata, the main site of cortisol production, and the zona reticularis, the main site of adrenal androgen production.

④ **A (corpus luteum)**
This is a bit of a sneaky question because you would have to remember that progesterone is thermogenic. This characteristic is important though, because it allows relatively accurate and straightforward identification of the time of ovulation due to a rise in core temperature.

⑤ **K (wolffian ducts)**
The wolffian ducts persist and develop into the male reproductive tract only in the presence of testosterone. The default position is the development of the mullerian ducts into the female reproductive tract.

⑥ **C (islets of Langerhans)**
The clusters of hormone secreting cells make up only about 2% of the mass of the pancreas. There are four main cell types in the islet producing insulin, glucagon, somatostatin and pancreatic polypeptide.

Endocrine cells I
① **A (acidophil cells)**
Hormone secreting cells of the anterior pituitary are divided into acidophil and basophil cells, according to their histological staining properties. The acidophil cells include somatotrophs and lactotrophs.

② **L (Sertoli cells)**
Although the Leydig cells are the main endocrine part of the testis, Sertoli cells secrete the two peptides, activin and inhibin, which may have a role in feedback regulation.

③ **J (granulosa cells)**
Granulosa cells are the main steroid secreting cells in the ovary between days 1 and 14 of the cycle, after which the corpus luteum becomes more important.

④ **B (α cells)**
The α cells of the endocrine pancreas are less numerous than β cells and produce glucagon in response to low blood glucose levels.

⑤ **F (chief cells)**
Chief cells are the endocrine cells of the parathyroid glands.

⑥ **H (G cells)**
G cells are found in the antral portion of the gastric mucosa. Gastrin stimulates gastric acid and pepsin secretion.

Endocrine cells II
① **F (chief cells)**
This is an example of a homeostatic mechanism. Low calcium concentration stimulates PTH secretion by chief cells and this tends to raise plasma calcium. High calcium levels inhibit PTH secretion, tending to lower plasma calcium levels.

② **D (β cells)**
The combination of GLUT2 and glucokinase is not a classical 'receptor', like the insulin receptor, but it functions in the same way. It detects increases in blood glucose levels and sends an intracellular signal to bring about insulin secretion.

③ **K (Leydig cells)**
Both pituitary basophil cells, which produce LH and FSH, and Sertoli cells are necessary for spermatogenesis; it is only testosterone secreted by Leydig cells that has a paracrine effect. Testosterone produced by the Leydig cells diffuses within the testis to the Sertoli cells without requiring circulation in the blood.

④ **E (C cells)**
These are also known as thyroid parafollicular cells and produce calcitonin. Absence of calcitonin appears to cause no ill effect and its only possible role seems to be in pregnancy.

⑤ **A (acidophil cells)**
Both somatotrophs and lactotrophs have cell surface dopamine receptors. Only the lactotrophs are under tonic inhibitory regulation by dopamine, but inhibition of somatotrophs by dopamine is used therapeutically

to shrink growth hormone producing adenomas using dopamine agonist drugs such as bromocriptine.

⑥ J (granulosa cells)
The early steps in the steroid biosynthetic path in the ovary take place in theca cells. Oestradiol is produced mainly in the granulosa cells by conversion from thecal androgens using the enzyme aromatase.

Hormonal secretion
① D (ectopic secretion)
Ectopic secretion means production of a hormone by a tissue that does not normally produce it. As well as small cell carcinomas of the lung, pancreatic islet cell carcinomas occasionally secrete ACTH. In both cases the result is Cushing's syndrome.

② J (paracrine effect)
A paracrine effect describes the action of a hormone on a different cell type in the same organ in which it was produced. Sertoli cells are arranged in proximity to Leydig cells within the testis.

③ E (endocrine effect)
Testosterone, secreted by the testis, can reach the brain only via the circulation. This is a classical endocrine effect. Testosterone influences many aspects of behaviour by its actions on the brain.

④ G (exocytosis)
Preformed insulin is stored in secretory granules in the β cells. These granules fuse with the cell membrane to release their contents when the β cells are stimulated.

⑤ L (simple diffusion)
All steroid hormones are lipid soluble and can diffuse passively across cell membranes.

⑥ I (neuroendocrine secretion)
Both of the posterior pituitary hormones, AVP and oxytocin, are produced in the hypothalamus and travel down neuronal projections into the posterior pituitary. They are released directly from these nerve endings into the circulation.

Note: In case you wondered, apocrine secretion, for example from the sweat glands, was so called because it used to be believed that the secretion was produced by breakdown of the gland's cells. Phagocytosis refers to the process of ingestion by cells of other cells, fragments of tissue and foreign bodies.

Concepts in endocrinology
① H (negative feedback)
Negative feedback allows both fine tuning and responsiveness within an endocrine axis. For example, within the hypothalamo–pituitary–gonadal axis there are multiple layers of feedback. Classically, negative feedback involves inhibition of a hypothalamic or pituitary peptide by the hormonal product of the end-organ of the cascade.

② I (neuroendocrine reflex)
This is the classical example of a neuroendocrine reflex. During lactation, suckling stimulates sensory nerves from the nipple. The signal is relayed to the hypothalamus and from there to the posterior pituitary, causing release of oxytocin.

③ L (synergistic action)
Many hormones have additive effects but relatively few have synergistic effects. The classical example of endocrine synergy is CRH and AVP acting together to increase ACTH secretion greatly.

④ C (diurnal variation)
Many hormones have characteristic and predictable patterns of secretion through the day. For example, melatonin is produced mainly at night. ACTH secretion, on the other hand, is lowest at around midnight, reaches a peak at about 6–7 am and gradually declines throughout the day, with small peaks at meal-times.

⑤ D (dynamic test)
Dynamic tests are particularly useful when investigating a deficiency or excess of a hormone. Growth hormone secretion is normally switched off by increased blood glucose levels, so failure of raised growth hormone secretion to suppress during a glucose tolerance test indicates an adenoma.

⑥ G (homeostatic mechanism)
There are many other examples of homeostatic mechanisms within the body, for example maintenance of blood sodium, potassium and calcium levels. Many of these are under endocrine control.

Named disorders
① C (Cushing's syndrome)
Any state of glucocorticoid excess, whether caused by endogenous or exogenous glucocorticoid, is known as Cushing's syndrome. Cushing's disease refers specifically to a pituitary adenoma that produces excess ACTH.

② K (Turner's syndrome)
The usual karyotype for Turner's syndrome is XO. In addition to the features in the question, Turner's syndrome results in abnormalities of the cardiovascular system. Although it affects 1 in 2000 newborn girls, the majority of fetuses with this abnormality are miscarried.

③ F (Klinefelter's syndrome)
The usual karyotype for Klinefelter's syndrome is XXY, although there may be even more extra copies of the

X chromosome. About 1 in 800 newborn boys is affected.

④ **G (Kussmaul's respiration)**
This is the deep, sighing respiration characteristic of diabetic ketoacidosis. It represents the body's attempt to maintain homeostasis by excreting more carbon dioxide in an attempt to raise blood pH.

⑤ **L (Zollinger–Ellison syndrome)**
This memorably named syndrome refers to the intractable peptic ulceration caused by the excess gastric acid associated with a gastrin-secreting tumour.

⑥ **H (Laron's syndrome)**
Don't be put off by the occasional question that refers to 'small print' knowledge. Very often, a set of six extended matching questions will have two easy ones, two or three moderately difficult ones, and one or two that are hard.

Note: Reaven's syndrome is one of the many synonyms for the metabolic syndrome (syndrome X, insulin resistance syndrome).

Drugs and hormones I: therapeutic uses
① **C (bromocriptine)**
Bromocriptine can also be used to shrink growth hormone secreting adenomas as both acidophil cell types have surface dopamine receptors.

② **E (carbimazole)**
Carbimazole inhibits thyroperoxidase activity and can be used either to control symptoms of thyrotoxicosis or to help reduce the size of the gland prior to surgery.

③ **I (metformin)**
Metformin is the only biguanide in the list. Sulphonylureas are also used in the management of NIDDM owing to their effect on stimulating insulin secretion. Metformin acts by a variety of mechanisms, mostly unclear.

④ **F (desmopressin)**
Conventional wisdom is that peptide hormones have to be injected to have any effect. However, desmopressin was the first peptide to be used therapeutically via the intranasal route. This requires larger doses than would be given by injection. Some peptides, in very large doses, are even active orally (like desmopressin).

⑤ **K (statin)**
Raised levels of cholesterol are characteristic of the metabolic syndrome and can be reduced by the statin family of drugs. Metformin is also used in the management of the metabolic syndrome but is not a HMG CoA reductase inhibitor.

⑥ **A (ACE inhibitor)**
The full name gives it away, as angiotensin converting enzyme inhibitors act on the renin–angiotensin system to reduce angiotensin II and aldosterone levels.

Drugs and hormones II: adverse effects
① **G (NSAID)**
Non-steroidal anti-inflammatory drugs inhibit cyclo-oxygenase systems. As a result, there is a theoretical impairment of ovulation, owing to the fact that prostaglandins are essential in this process.

② **D (chlorpropamide)**
This potential adverse effect can be used to therapeutic advantage in the management of nephrogenic diabetes insipidus.

③ **C (chlorpromazine)**
Chlorpromazine is a traditional antipsychotic drug whose therapeutic effects are due to central dopamine antagonism. This can also affect the anterior pituitary resulting in raised prolactin levels.

④ **B (carbamazepine)**
It is a source of constant irritation to medical students and doctors that drug chemists come up with such similar names for different drugs. Carbamazepine, chlorpromazine and chlorpropamide are a good example of how easy it is to get confused.

⑤ **J (stanozolol)**
Stanozolol is a synthetic anabolic androgenic steroid (AAS). It is commonly abused by athletes and body builders owing to the increased muscle bulk that it promotes, but infertility is only one of many adverse effects. In more sophisticated steroid-abusing regimes, β-hCG is given at the end of the anabolic steroid cycle in order to restore the hypothalamo–pituitary testicular axis and prevent testicular atrophy.

⑥ **H (prednisolone)**
Prednisolone is a potent synthetic glucocorticoid often used in the management of inflammatory disorders. High doses of prednisolone can cause depression and, more commonly, elated mood states.

Drugs and hormones III: the adrenals
① **F (glycerrhitinic acid)**
This is the reason why eating excessive amounts of liquorice can cause the disorder 'apparent mineralocorticoid excess'.

② **G (hydrocortisone)**
Cortisol and hydrocortisone are identical, but cortisol refers to the naturally occurring hormone and hydrocortisone to the drug.

③ **E (dexamethasone)**

Other synthetic glucocorticoids, such as prednisolone, have some mineralocorticoid activity. Hydrocortisone (cortisol) has sufficient mineralocorticoid activity that it can be given on its own as a replacement therapy after bilateral adrenalectomy.

④ **L (spironolactone)**

Clinically, spironolactone is used as a potassium-sparing diuretic owing to its blockade of aldosterone receptors. It can also be used to treat Conn's syndrome, a rare disorder of mineralocorticoid excess.

⑤ **H (phenoxybenzamine)**

Phenoxybenzamine is the only α-adrenergic antagonist in the list. Propranolol and atenolol are both β-adrenergic receptor antagonists. In the treatment of phaeochromocytoma, α blockade is always started before β blockade.

⑥ **C (dehydroepiandrosterone)**

Better known in its abbreviated form, DHEA, this is the major product of the human adrenal cortex but does not have a clearly defined role.

Endocrine investigation

① **C (dexamethasone suppression test)**

Because dexamethasone is not detected by standard cortisol assays, it can be given orally and followed by blood tests for cortisol. A normal result is suppression of cortisol due to negative feedback by dexamethasone on the HPA axis. Failure to suppress is an abnormal result and suggests autonomous HPA activity (e.g. in the presence of a tumour).

② **H (MIBG scan)**

This radioisotope is taken up by catecholamine-producing tissues and enables visualization of the location of phaeochromocytomas. This is particularly useful when they are ectopic (outside the adrenal medulla).

③ **G (insulin tolerance test)**

Normally, inducing hypoglycaemia by injecting insulin (under very controlled conditions – don't try this at home) stimulates the production of GH and ACTH. In hypopituitarism, growth hormone, and later ACTH, fails to respond.

④ **F (heel-prick blood test)**

This test is simple to perform, usually at 1 week of age, and allows the prevention of a devastating disorder. Congenital hypothyroidism affects about 1 in 4000 children born in the UK and, if left untreated, results in profound intellectual and developmental impairment (cretinism).

⑤ **A (chromosomal analysis)**

Chromosomal analysis reveals a person's karyotype, which may be different from their physical appearance or phenotype. The most common cause of primary hypogonadism is Klinefelter's syndrome (47XXY), which affects around 1 in 800 baby boys.

⑥ **K (urinary hCG immunoassay)**

Allowing earlier detection of pregnancy than the toad bioassay, urinary hCG immunoassay is now the standard pregnancy test. Home testing kits have a built-in colour change to signify a positive result, whereas laboratory testing will give a quantitative measure of the amount of hormone. This allows detection of the rare and non-viable abnormality of pregnancy known as hydatidiform mole, which produces large amounts of hCG. Because the α-chain of hCG is identical to the α-chain of TSH, hydatidiform mole is also associated with the features of thyrotoxicosis.

Endocrine biochemistry

① **F (raised calcium level in blood)**

PTHrp produced by tumours has the same effect as PTH and raises blood calcium levels.

② **E (low sodium level in blood)**

Renin release by the kidney is stimulated by low blood sodium levels and reduced renal perfusion (hypotension or hypovolaemia).

③ **D (low potassium level in blood)**

Mineralocorticoids stimulate sodium reabsorption with the loss of potassium.

④ **I (raised glucose level in blood)**

HbA1c is glycated haemoglobin and correlates with average blood glucose levels over the previous few weeks.

⑤ **G (high cholesterol level in blood)**

The metabolic syndrome is also associated with raised blood glucose levels, but only raised cholesterol concentration is reduced by treatment with statins. It is the concentration of triglycerides that is raised in the metabolic syndrome, not that of free fatty acids.

⑥ **C (low pH level in blood)**

This is associated with diabetic ketoacidosis, owing to the rise in levels of free fatty acids.

Hormone deficiency

① **H (insulin)**

This is the classical presentation of insulin-dependent diabetes mellitus.

② **D (erythropoietin)**

Chronic renal failure may be associated with deficiency of erythropoietin, a hormone produced by the kidney that stimulates red blood cell production in the bone marrow.

③ **J (parathyroid hormone)**
The parathyroid glands are often embedded in thyroid tissue and may all be removed in a total thyroidectomy. The result is hypocalcaemia, which causes tetany, a hypersensitivity of muscle fibres, and tingling in fingers and lips.

④ **K (testosterone)**
Orchitis is inflammation of the testes, and mumps can be a very nasty illness in adult men. It is a recognized cause, along with radiation and chemotherapy, of acquired primary hypogonadism.

⑤ **L (thyroxine)**
This question is a good example of how extended matching questions (EMQs) differ from multiple choice questions (MCQs). If the MCQ was 'Could low thyroxine levels explain these findings in a woman taking lithium?', you would need to know that lithium can cause hypothyroidism. In an EMQ you know the statement is true, so you don't need to know that lithium causes hypothyroidism, just that the description is the classical presentation of thyroxine deficiency.

⑥ **B (cortisol)**
High doses of glucocorticoids, taken as drugs, suppress the HPA axis. If the exogenous steroid is stopped suddenly, it takes a long time for the axis to recover and may result in acute adrenal insufficiency, or addisonian crisis. The situation is exacerbated by stress, which normally triggers increased HPA activity.

Hormone excess
① **G (oxytocin)**
The only known physiological roles for oxytocin are in the suckling reflex and parturition. There is no syndrome of excess oxytocin secretion.

② **A (ACTH)**
This is the classical description of Cushing's syndrome, which can be due to an excess of ACTH resulting in raised cortisol levels.

③ **E (GH)**
This is another classical description, this time of acromegaly.

④ **D (adrenaline)**
Excess adrenaline (epinephrine) is produced by phaeochromocytomas. Some of the effects may also be seen in thyrotoxicosis, for example caused by raised TSH. However, adrenaline antagonizes insulin and, like GH and ACTH, an excess is associated with impaired glucose tolerance. Adrenaline also causes dilatation of the pupil.

⑤ **H (prolactin)**
Very high levels of prolactin in men, due to a prolactinoma or adverse drug effects, may be associated with gynaecomastia and even milk production.

⑥ **L (VIP)**
Vasoactive intestinal polypeptide can be produced in excessive amounts by VIPomas, resulting in a characteristic presentation.

And finally…
① **D (gadfly)**
Oestrous is a period of sexual receptivity.

② **B (cow)**
Pigs also have only one oestrous cycle per year.

③ **C (dog)**
Only higher primates have menstrual cycles with regular bleeding but many animals are continuous cyclers (e.g. rat).

④ **L (toad)**
Specifically the clawed toad, *Xenopus laevis*.

⑤ **K (salmon)**
Salmon calcitonin can be used as an injection or nasal spray in the treatment of osteoporosis and Paget's disease for patients who do not tolerate bisphosphonates.

⑥ **H (lizard)**
Lerner discovered melatonin in 1958 in his search for the hormone that controls skin colour change in lizards.

GLOSSARY

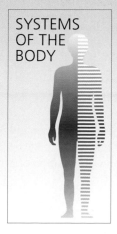

SYSTEMS
OF THE
BODY

AII – angiotensin II.

AAS – anabolic androgenic steroids.

ABP – androgen binding protein, found in the testes.

ACE – angiotensin converting enzyme.

ACTH – adrenocorticotropic hormone = corticotropin.

ADH – anti-diuretic hormone = AVP.

AME – apparent mineralocorticoid excess.

AMH – anti-mullerian hormone.

ANP – atrial natriuretic peptide.

aquaporin 2 – a protein on the apical membrane of cells lining the renal collecting ducts whose production is stimulated by AVP. This protein functions as a water channel.

autocrine – when the hormone acts locally, on the same type of cell that produces it.

AVP – arginine vasopressin.

bioassay – a method for measuring hormones based on the biological response they produce.

BMI – body mass index, calculated by: weight (kg)/height squared (metres).

cAMP – cyclic adenosine monophosphate (a second messenger).

CBG – cortisol binding globulin = transcortin.

CCK – cholecystokinin.

cGMP – cyclic guanosine monophosphate.

climacteric – the period of time, which includes the menopause, when a woman's menstrual cycle becomes irregular and ceases, as a result of age.

COX – cyclo-oxygenase, enzymes involved in prostaglandin synthesis.

C-peptide – the connecting peptide, which is cleaved from the A- and B-peptides comprising mature insulin, and released into the circulation with insulin.

CRH – corticotropin releasing hormone.

CT – computed tomography, a scanning X-ray that can build up a two-dimensional slice picture or, with software, a three-dimensional image.

Cushing's disease – a condition of glucocorticoid excess caused by ACTH secretion from a pituitary tumour.

Cushing's syndrome – the symptoms of glucocorticoid excess, due to any cause, including the use of corticosteroids as a medicine.

CYP – a gene family that encodes the cytochrome P450 hydroxylase enzymes involved in steroid biosynthesis.

DAG – diacylglycerol.

DBP – vitamin D binding protein.

desmopressin – synthetic analogue of arginine vasopressin that can be administered orally or by nasal spray.

DHEA(S) – dehydroepiandrosterone (sulphate), the most abundant androgen secreted by the adrenal cortex.

DHT – 5α-dihydrotestosterone.

diurnal variation – the predictable daily pattern of secretion of a hormone.

dynamic test – the measurement of a hormone in response to an agent that normally either stimulates or suppresses its secretion.

ectopic hormone secretion – the inappropriate secretion of a hormone by a tissue that does not usually produce it.

EGF – epidermal growth factor.

endocrine – secretion of hormones directly into the bloodstream by a ductless tissue.

EPO – erythropoietin.

exocrine – secretion of the product of a gland via a secretory duct.

FFAs – free fatty acids.

FSH – follicle stimulating hormone.

GFR – glomerular filtration rate.

GH – growth hormone.

GHRH – growth hormone releasing hormone.

glucocorticoid – a class of steroid produced by the adrenal cortex that binds to the intracellular glucocorticoid (cortisol) receptor and has a role in the regulation of metabolism.

GLUT – a family of glucose transporter proteins.

GnRH – gonadotropin releasing hormone.

G protein – guanyl nucleotide binding protein.

HbA1c – glycated haemoglobin, a measure of 'average' blood glucose concentration.

hCG – human chorionic gonadotropin.

HDL – high-density lipoprotein.

HLA gene – human leucocyte antigen, a histocompatability locus gene.

HPA axis – hypothalamo–pituitary–adrenal axis.

hPL – human placental lactogen.

HRE – hormone response element. An area in the promoter region of a gene that allows hormones to stimulate or repress gene transcription.

HRT – hormone replacement therapy.

hsp – heat shock proteins (associated with steroid receptors in the resting state).

hydrocortisone – the name given to cortisol when it is used therapeutically.

IDDM – type 1 diabetes mellitus (insulin-dependent diabetes mellitus).

IGF – insulin-like growth factor.

IP$_3$ – inositol trisphosphate, a second messenger.

IRS – not the inland revenue service, but insulin receptor substrate.

JAK–STAT – Janus-associated kinase–signal transducer and activator of transcription.

kinase – an enzyme that catalyses the phosphorylation of a substrate protein.

LDL – low-density lipoprotein.

LH – luteinizing hormone.

MAPK – mitogen-activated protein kinase.

MEN – multiple endocrine neoplasia.

menarche – a girl's first menstrual period.

menopause – permanent cessation of menstruation, defined as 12 months since the last monthly period.

mineralocorticoid – a class of steroid hormones secreted by the adrenal cortex that has a role in the regulation of salt balance.

MRI – magnetic resonance imaging.

NIDDM – type 2 diabetes mellitus (non-insulin-dependent diabetes mellitus).

NOS – nitric oxide synthase.

NSAIDs – non-steroidal anti-inflammatory drugs.

OGTT – oral glucose tolerance test.

osmolality – the number of osmoles per kilogram of solvent.

osmolarity – the number of osmoles per litre of solvent.

paracrine – when a hormone acts locally, within the same tissue, on a cell type that is different to the cell that secreted the hormone.

PCOS – polycystic ovarian syndrome.

PIP_2 – phosphatidylinositol bisphosphate.

PLA2 – phospholipase A2. An enzyme that converts membrane phospholipids to arachidonic acid; the first step in prostaglandin production.

plasma – whole blood that is prevented from clotting prior to centrifugation. Does not contain cells but does contain clotting factors.

PLC – phospholipase C. An enzyme involved in second messenger production.

PNMT – phenylethanolamine *n*-methyltransferase, the enzyme that catalyses the formation of adrenaline from noradrenaline.

polydipsia – excessive drinking (usually refers to non-alcoholic drinks!).

polyuria – the production of excessive quantities of urine.

POMC – pro-opio-melanocortin.

portal system – a vascular connection with two sets of capillary beds.

PRL (Prl) – prolactin.

PTH – parathyroid hormone.

PTHrp – parathyroid hormone-related peptide.

reverse T3 – thyroxine that has had one iodine residue removed, producing an inactive hormone.

serum – the liquid component of blood without the cells, obtained by allowing whole blood to clot, then centrifuging the clot (including cells) away from the serum.

SHBG – sex hormone binding globulin.

SIADH – syndrome of inappropriate anti-diuretic hormone.

SRY – sex-determining region Y (testis determining factor).

StAR – steroidogenic acute regulatory protein.

T3 – thyroxine that has had one iodine residue removed, producing an active hormone.

T4 – thyroxine, thyroid hormone.

TeBG – testosterone binding globulin = SHBG.

TGFβ – transforming growth factor β.

THBG – thyroid hormone binding globulin.

thyrotoxicosis – the clinical disease state caused by excess thyroid hormone.

TK – tyrosine kinase.

TRH – thyrotropin releasing hormone.

tropic hormones – hormones that regulate other endocrine glands.

TSH – thyroid stimulating hormone = thyrotropin.

VIP – vasoactive intestinal polypeptide.

INDEX

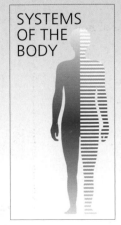

SYSTEMS
OF THE
BODY

Page numbers in *italics* refer to figures and tables.